Parents, Families, and the Stuttering Child

Far Communication Disorders Series

Series Editors: Chris Code and David Rowley, Department of Speech Pathology, Leicester Polytechnic, Leicester, England.

The *Far Communication Disorders Series* aims to provide books in speech and language pathology and therapy for the clinician and student clinician. Each book in the series will aim to be practical, readable and affordable. Currently available and forthcoming titles include:

Parents, Families, and the Stuttering Child
Edited by Lena Rustin

Treating Phonological Disorders in Children. Metaphon - Theory to Practice
Janet Howell & Elizabeth Dean

Assessment and Management of Emotional and Psychosocial Reactions to Aphasia and Brain Damage
Peter Währborg

Group Encounters in Communication Disorders
Edited by Margaret Fawcus

Management of Acquired Aphasia in Children
Janet Lees

The Clinician's Guide to Linguistic Profiling of Language Impairment
Martin J Ball

Cluttering: A Clinical Perspective
Edited by Florence Myers & Kenneth O St Louis

Computers in Management and Therapy
Edited by David Rowley & Chris Code

Introductory Guide to Clinical Syntactic Analysis
Eeva Leinonen & Susan Fasler

Which Screen? A User's Guide to Speech and Language Screening Tests
Joanne Corcoran

Parents, Families, and the Stuttering Child

Edited by Lena Rustin

SINGULAR PUBLISHING GROUP, INC.
SAN DIEGO, CALIFORNIA

Copyright 1991 by **Far Communications Ltd.**, 5 Harcourt Estate, Kibworth, Leics. LE7 0NE, **Great Britain.**

British Library Cataloguing in Publication Data:
Parents, Families, and the stuttering child.
1. Speech disorders
I. Rustin, Lena
618.92855406

ISBN 0 9514728-4-4

Published and Distributed in the United States and Canada by
Singular Publishing Group Inc.,
4284 41st. St.,
San Diego,
California 92105

ISBN 1-879105-16-0

Printed and Bound in Great Britain by
BPCC Wheatons Ltd., Exeter.

CONTENTS

PREFACE

The seeds of an idea for this book were planted at the 2nd Oxford Disfluency Conference which took place in August 1989. Contributors from many countries presented papers on research and management of childhood disfluency and we were most grateful to Travers Reid, Chairman of the Association for Research into Stammering in Childhood for a substantial contribution towards getting the conference off the ground.

This book is concerned with the role of parents and families in the management of stuttering, an area which has received little attention in the past. Chapters 1 presents discussion on the major factors to emerge from analysis of a large database of information collected on families of stuttering children and Chapter 2 reviews the relevance of speech production to the management of the stuttering child.

Chapters 3, 4 and 5 are concerned with the nature of the interactions between pre-school and school age children and their families, and the changes that can be implemented. Chapters 6 and 7 address the issues which are particularly relevant to the management of adolescent stutterers.

My aims were to make this book practical, readable and attractive to clinicians and students working with children and adolescents with fluency problems. I am grateful to the contributors for helping me achieve those aims. As authors are from both sides of the Atlantic, they have used their own native English spelling conventions in their chapters.

LR
20 February 1991

CONTRIBUTORS

Willie Botterill, Speech Therapy Service, Finsbury Health Centre, Pine St., London EC1R 0JH, United Kingdom.

Edward G. Conture, Communication Disorders and Sciences, Syracuse University, 805 South Crouse Avenue, Syracuse, New York 13244-2280, U.S.A.

Frances Cook, Speech Therapy Service, Finsbury Health Centre, Pine St., London EC1R 0JH, United Kingdom.

Carolyn B. Gregory, Private Practice Specialist in Stuttering Therapy, 2400 Brown Avenue, Evanston, Illinois 60201, U.S.A.

Hugo H. Gregory, Professor & Director or Stuttering Programs, Department of Communication Sciences and Disorders, Northwestern University, Evanston, Illinois 6020, U.S.A.

Ellen M. Kelly, Department of Audiology and Speech Sciences, Purdue University, West Lafayette, Indiana 47907, U.S.A.

Elaine Kelman, Speech Therapy Service, Finsbury Health Centre, Pine St., London EC1R 0JH, United Kingdom.

A. R. Mallard, Director, Communication Disorders Program, School of Health Professions, Southwest Texas State University, San Marcos, TX 78666-4616, USA.

Susan C Meyers, Associate Professor, Department of Communicative Disorders, California State University, Northridge, 18111 Nordhoff St., Northridge, CA 91330, USA.

Harry Purser, Director of Planning and Contracting, Bloomsbury, Islington and Hampstead Health Authority, London, United Kingdom.

Lena Rustin, District Speech Therapist, Bloomsbury, Islington and Hampstead Health Authority, Speech Therapy Service, Finsbury Health Centre, Pine St., London EC1R 0JH, United Kingdom.

Chapter 1

Child Development, Families, and the Problem of Stuttering

Lena Rustin and Harry Purser

Introduction

In this chapter the preliminary findings from a survey aimed at studying the developmental history and family circumstances of children who stutter are presented. Whilst there have been numerous studies undertaken to date which have examined the relationship between stuttering and key aspects of development, such as language acquisition, motor development, and educational progress, (see Andrews *et al* 1983 for a comprehensive review), there have been relatively few which have adopted a single case study approach to cataloguing the general developmental history of children who stutter. In the sections that follow we describe some of the findings that have emerged from such an approach to the study of childhood disfluency involving over 200 individual case histories.

The work described here was undertaken within the context of Rustin's (1989) approach to the assessment and treatment of disfluent children and their families. Rustin has developed a structured interview protocol as a central component of the assessment process which systematically probes for data about key events occurring during development and the family systems within which development takes place. A large part of this interview protocol is reproduced in the appendix at the end of this chapter. Both parents participate in the interview answering questions about their child's general developmental history together with his current behaviour and affective state. The interview also focuses on family relationships in order to obtain a flavour of the wider context within which the disfluent child is developing.

Information gathered through the structured parental interview is then classified using an empirically reliable coding system. The basis of this classification system is the detection of clinically significant problems. The coded information is then entered on a computerised database system for cumulative analysis. To date this database contains the details of over 200 cases treated through Rustin's **Child and Family** programme.

1

In the sections that follow a number of areas of child development are explored through the analysis of 209 completed case histories. The overall conclusion which emerges from this analysis is that the disfluent children included in this study exhibit much higher problem rates, of both an individual and family nature, than would otherwise be expected given their age and social background. If this conclusion applies to the general population of stutterers there are many implications for the assessment and treatment of disfluent children and their families. However, the possibility exists that the sample of stuttering children studied here may not be fully representative of the general population of disfluent children and families. The children referred to the speech therapy department are largely *tertiary referrals*. In the majority of cases the referrer is another speech clinician and the general impression is that these referrals have a tendency to be the more difficult cases for whom a two week intensive programme of fluency therapy is indicated. Therefore, there is the distinct possibility that the data obtained from this sample may only tell us something about the sub-population of *more severe and more persistent* fluency problems.

Bearing these points in mind we can now turn to the analysis of the database itself, and the findings we obtained about the developmental history of children with persistent disfluency.

The Sample

Data were gathered over a period of three years on a sample of 209 children who were assessed on the Rustin (1987) interview procedure. The referrals in the main came from speech therapists in the South East of England. However, some cases were drawn from the local population served by the Bloomsbury, Hampstead and Islington speech therapy services and many of these were direct GP referrals. All children were referred for full consultation and both parents had to attend. The fluency problem itself had to be sufficiently severe to warrant inclusion in the programme, and in this context parental judgement of severity was considered the most significant indicator of handicapping disfluency.

The average age of the children included in the sample was 8.4 years with 18% of the children being aged under five years, 70% between 5 years and 13 years, and the remaining 12% over 13 years. There were 163 boys in the sample and 46 girls yielding a sex ratio of 3.5:1 [male:female], which is in line with the available epidemiological findings (Andrews *et al* 1983). The average age at onset of stuttering was 3 years 6 months with 27% of the sample reporting onset under three years, 68% between three years and seven years and the remaining 5% at 7 years and above. These statistics are again in line with current knowledge of the natural history of stuttering (Andrews and Harris 1964). Thus in terms of age distribution, sex ratio and age at onset the sample studied here conforms to the known parameters of childhood disfluency.

The Parental Interview

The starting point for parental involvement is the completion of the structured interview procedure which is administered by a small group of specially trained fluency therapists. The **Structured Parental Interview** evolved from existing assessment materials drawn from the fields of clinical psychology, child development and standard medical examination. The interview procedure itself is controlled through the use of a protocol which specifies standard probes for each area of development and lays down criteria for seeking clarification of particular points. The recording of the interview is achieved through clinician notes, often supplemented by audiotape, which are then coded as soon as possible after the interview is completed. Generally the child is assessed for cognitive abilities and fluency performance whilst the parents are undertaking the interview procedure.

The interview lasts between 120 and 180 minutes on average; coding the responses and highlighting specific areas generally takes a further 60 minutes. There is little doubt it is a time consuming activity; however, for a maximum of 4 hours of professional time per case, a very considerable amount of detailed clinical information can be obtained. In our experience there are many instances where the interview procedure itself has led to the immediate identification of specific problems which have subsequently been addressed within the therapy setting. We have no doubts about the value of the interview in relation to individual cases; the value of the cumulative database lies in its capacity to determine the **rates** of particular problems within this population. Given the high degree of professional effort that goes into eliciting and coding developmental information supplied by willing parents, some confidence can be placed in the analyses that emerge from the cumulative database. In the following sections some of the main findings are highlighted.

General Health

One of the earliest questions asked of parents in the interview procedure is the extent to which their child has been consistently missing time at school for frequent or recurrent general health problems in the previous twelve months. Only 3.7% of the sample confirmed such a systematic pattern of poor general health. However, a further 15% of the parents reported that there had been significant periods in their child's development where marked and persistent ill health (i.e. beyond simple childhood disorders such as mumps, measles, etc) had been experienced and had interfered significantly with schooling.

Parents are also asked to describe any health problems affecting their disfluent child where secondary hospital treatment has been necessary. In all 76% of the boys and 65% of the girls in the sample had experienced either an in-patient hospital stay of one night or more, or a series of outpatient consultations for a specific health problem. Half the boys in the sample had been admitted to hospital as an in-patient at some point in development and 29% of the girls. A further quarter of the boys and over one third of the girls in the sample had attended non speech pathology hospital outpatient clinics. These rates appear well above expectation and point to the existence of acute as well as persistent general health difficulties within the sample.

In all some 222 individual medical problems were detected in the sample which were distributed amongst 72 children, just over one third of the sample. Around 42% of the 72 children had **one** significant medical problem; a further 42% had **two** significant problems, and 15% had **three** problems in coexistence. A small number of children (<1%) had four or more problems coexisting.

Table 1 shows the proportion of the problems distributed between each of six categories. Recurrent abdominal pain made up the single largest problem category. The overall rate of significant health problems in the sample runs at 35%, an unexpectedly high proportion, but this figure covers a wide age range. Further analyses need to be undertaken to establish the age-specific problem rates. The overall prevalence rates for these problems in the sample are also shown in Table 1. Each problem has a much higher prevalence in this sample of disfluent children than would be expected in a comparable cohort of fluent children. Although the number of females in the sample is relatively small, there are some very interesting sex differences in the rates for each of the main problem categories. For example, the rate for asthma is roughly twice as high in girls as in boys, though the rate for recurrent **headaches** in girls is half that seen in boys. Sight and hearing problems were found to be twice as high in boys.

TABLE 1 Physical Symptoms

CONDITION	Frequency (N=222 problems in 72 children - 35% of the sample)	Overall Prevalence in the sample (N=209 children)
Asthma	11%	11%
Headaches	15%	16%
Abdominal pains	21%	22%
Sight	17%	18%
Hearing	13%	14%
Other (allergies, infections, etc)	23%	24%
Total	100%	N/A

In another section of the interview the existence of further difficulties in sleeping, eating and elimination was examined. The majority of these problems are age-related and parents were asked whether they considered their disfluent child currently experienced marked problems in these areas relative to siblings and other children. Such symptoms are often associated with various forms of developmental disability and this analysis is shown for the entire sample in Table 2. Reports of poor appetite and food fads were obtained for 25% of the boys and nearly one third of the girls. The criterion for the recording of this type of problem here was that the problem had to be sufficiently severe or persistent to warrant an opinion from the child's general practitioner. Although none of the cases in the current sample were reported as displaying the classic signs of *anorexia nervosa*, there does seem to be a very high incidence of milder forms of eating disorders which is consistent with observations made by Bruch (1973).

Just over one third of the boys in the sample and one fifth of the girls were reported by their parents as having significant sleep problems in relation to their siblings. These ranged from an inability to get off to sleep at night to difficulty waking up in the mornings. By far the most common problem was of a restless child who wakes several times during the night. The American Association of Sleep Disorders Centers describe a group of sleep disorders which they term *parasomnias* that have been found to be particularly common in preschool and school-aged children (Anders 1980). Four separate disorders have been described: night terrors, sleepwalking, sleep talking and NREM-related enuresis. Using these criteria we recorded rates of sleepwalking of 6% amongst boys and 20% amongst girls

TABLE 2 Systems Problems

PROBLEM	BOYS	GIRLS
Eating	25%	32%
Sleeping	34%	23%
Sleepwalking	6%	20%
Nightmares	26%	20%
Enuresis	22%	9%

in the sample, though it is reported that up to 15% of normal children sleepwalk at least once. Night terrors (nightmares) affected 26% of boys and 20% of the girls compared with published norms of 1% to 4% in the general population.

Enuresis, as expected, was much higher in boys than in girls. However, this is an age-related problem where at 5 years some 14% of boys and girls wet at least once per month. By 7 years only 7% of boys and 3% of girls are affected and by 10 years this rate drops to 3% of boys and 2% of girls. One fifth of the boys in the sample were reported to be currently enuretic at night compared with 9% of the girls. Clearly this finding is well above expectation given the average age of the sample (8.4 years).

The relationship, if any, between these health problems and stuttering requires further investigation. Regardless of any direct relationships there will always be *indirect* effects through disruptions in schooling and relationships through ill health. With a base rate of nearly 20% of the children in this sample missing schooling for significant periods of time through ill health and a medical problem rate of 35% in the whole sample there is clearly a great deal of scope for this kind of disturbance in the course of development. Nevertheless, nearly two thirds of the sample did not suffer from significant health problems and the next

Child Development

part of the interview schedule probes for other kinds of difficulties which affect disfluent children.

Developmental History

Parents were asked to recall the ages at which the child reached various developmental milestones. Table 3 outlines the areas of development covered in this component of the interview. Gross motor development was assessed through parental recollection of the age at which the child began walking unaided.

TABLE 3 Developmental Milestones

3.1: Walking

SEX	< 12 months	13 - 18 months	19 months +
Boys	23%	40%	36%
Girls	27%	41%	32%

3.2: Language Development

SEX	SLOW	AVERAGE	ADVANCED
Boys	53%	20%	27%
Girls	46%	18%	36%

3.3: Clinic Attendances

SEX	Speech	Child Guidance	Other
Boys	92%	15%	14%
Girls	75%	7%	21%

This information is carefully elicited through cross-referencing to birthdays, Christmas and other memorable events. The rate of language development for each child was sought in relation to older and younger siblings. In the case of first or only children no data was elicited from parents for inclusion here (i.e. N=172 cases). Finally, attendances at various non-medical clinics (excluding speech clinics) were recorded.

Table 3.1 indicates a significant number of children walking rather later than would be expected from the usual norms and a high proportion of children (Table 3.2) were judged by their parents to be slow in their acquisition of language relative to their other siblings. Whilst this type of information is not *hard*, in that the information has been derived from a standardised assessment technique, it does indicate a marked perception amongst parents that their disfluent children are significantly slower than their siblings in general development.

Nearly all the boys in the sample had experienced contact with professional speech pathology services in the past (Table 3.3) and three quarters of the girls had received assessment and treatment for their fluency problem. This finding supports the notion that the majority of the sample was made up of tertiary referrals. The rate of Child Guidance clinic contact was 15% in boys and half that in girls. Attendances here were in the main for conduct and emotional problems. Both sexes show a significant rate of attendance at other specialist (non-medical) clinics such as Child Development Centres, primarily for specific concerns about the rate of overall development, though some parents did report these attendances were associated with fluency and speech development.

In the course of the developmental history taking parents were asked a number of specific questions about their child's usual level of functioning in particular areas. Parents reported 45% of boys and 36% of girls as being **overactive**, i.e. unable to sit quietly and concentrate on a task for some time. Parents described 23% of the boys and 45% of the girls as having poor concentration. One third of the boys were described as **clumsy** and **accident prone** against only 13% of the girls. These reports are consistent with general neuropsychological theories of disfluency (Moore & Boberg 1987) which imply generalised deficits in brain functioning leading to motor speech impulsivity and lack of neuromotor control (Rosenfield & Nudelman 1987). These symptoms are reminiscent of the *minimal brain dysfunction* concept (Clements 1966; Wender 1971; Rutter *et al* 1970) which implies a symptom complex of hyperactivity, emotionality, impulsivity and other soft neurological signs associated with attention, cognitive and learning deficits. Although the validity of the concept of *minimal brain*

Child Development

dysfunction is often held to be in question there is little doubt that parents do perceive a significant proportion of disfluent children as exhibiting the kinds of behavioural symptoms typically associated with the concept. Further, the usual sex differences in rates of such symptoms are less clear cut in the present sample than would be expected in a comparable group of children. Typically boys are reported to have a greater prevalence of these behavioural characteristics than girls.

Another popular hypothesis in relation to *minimal brain dysfunction*, and indeed neuropsychological disorders in general, concerns the prevalence of mixed handedness in positive samples. Handedness is viewed as a manifestation of cerebral lateralisation, with mixed handedness an indicator of incomplete or atypical neurological lateralisation. Table 4 indicates the assessed handedness of the children included in the present sample. The rates of right handedness are identical in both boys and girls, but there are marked differences in the incidence of left handedness between the sexes. This is almost twice as common in girls compared to boys, but boys are nearly twice as likely to demonstrate no particular preferred hand relative to girls. Here again, there may be no relationship between these findings and fluency problems in general, but it is conceivable that sub-groups of disfluent children exist where such findings are of etiological significance.

TABLE 4 Handedness

SEX	Right	Left	Mixed	Unknown
Boys	74%	6%	17%	3%
Girls	75%	11%	9%	5%

TABLE 5 Habit Disorders

SEX	Total of Sample	Facial Tics	Eye Blink	Thumb Sucking	Nail Biting	Soft Toy
Boys	35%	17%	10%	20%	33%	20%
Girls	27%	0 %	17%	41%	33%	8%

Finally, given the interest in stuttering as a **habit disorder** (Sheehan 1975; Shames & Sherrick 1963; Brutten & Shoemaker 1967) parents were asked to describe any specific habitual forms of behaviour their children engaged in. Table 5 outlines the findings in this section of the interview. Many forms of habitual behaviour are age-specific; in general such behaviours are common in younger children. It is only at later stages in development that such behaviours are defined as problems. Parents, upon reporting particular habitual mannerisms, were asked if, given the age of their child, they considered the behaviour problematic and whether they would want to pursue treatment for their children.

In this sample in over a third of the boys and more than a quarter of the girls there was evidence of clear cut habit disorders, even when developmental level was taken into account. Seventeen percent of the boys in the sample were described by their parents as having marked facial tics. This type of problem was non-existent amongst females, though they were reported as having a higher proportion of eyeblinking behaviour than the boys. Thumb sucking was found to be a particularly significant problem in females. More boys than girls continued to have attachments to a particular soft toy at ages where such attachments are usually rare. Again, many children had more than one habit problem in coexistence; the percentages in Table 5 for each problem category relate to the overall frequency of each individual problem in the subsample.

The extent to which these types of problems are related to stuttering is difficult to establish. In the minds of many parents in the sample a relationship was implied, particularly for facial and eyelid mannerisms which were almost invariably reported as concomitant with speech disfluency. Other habits, such as thumb sucking, nail biting and attachments to soft toys were viewed by parents as being associated with their child's emotional state (see below). Stuttering was therefore being used as an explanation for these habits.

Current Behaviour

The structured interview procedure places considerable emphasis on eliciting information about the child's current behavioural, emotional and social functioning. Many theories of disfluency have rounded on both **emotional** and **social** functioning as a partial explanation for the development of disfluency. It is therefore of interest to note the descriptions offered by parents of their child's typical functioning in these areas.

Child Development

Emotional Functioning

Parents were first asked how they would characterise their stuttering child overall. Some 7% of parents found this opening question too general to answer but 85% of parents described their child as generally happy and apparently content. Some 8% of parents described their child as appearing miserable and unhappy a great deal of the time. Both sexes were described as being prone to frequent crying sessions (16% of sample).

Parents were asked whether they thought their child **worried** excessively about events. Some 44% of the sample were described by their parents as definitely having worries about a wide range of events and specific situations. Forty-three percent of the boys and half the girls in the sample were described by their parents as being fastidious and fussy about their possessions, clothes, and other aspects of their life in the family.

Table 6 outlines parental responses to questions about the predominant affective characteristics of their disfluent children. Once again, many children were described as falling into more than one category, thus the percentages shown represent the proportion of parents identifying each characteristic in their child.

TABLE 6 Child Emotional Behaviour

SEX	Irritable	Sulks	Temper Tantrums	School Refusal
Boys	42%	30%	52%	5.5%
Girls	30%	25%	36%	9%

The children in this sample show high perceived rates of negative emotional expression. The incidence of **school refusal** (Hersov 1960, 1977) was far higher in girls than in boys. In general populations the prevalence of school refusal is between 1% and 5% depending on age. In this sample boys attained the high end of this range, but the rate was twice as high in girls. A significant proportion of boys, some 52%, were described by their parents as prone to extreme and inconsolable **temper tantrums** at various times. Over 40% of the boys were reported by their parents as showing inappropriate **irritability**, both with adults and with other children. Nearly a third of the girls in this sample were similarly described by their parents.

Social Functioning

Many pioneers of fluency treatment have sought the secret of stuttering in the development of social relationships. The interview technique explores the social functioning of stuttering children to arrive at a picture of the child's relationships both with their siblings and peers, and indeed with the parents themselves. This section of the interview is approached towards the end of the session in order that parents feel sufficiently secure and relaxed to answer the questions fully and frankly. Half the children in the sample were described by their parents as getting on well with their peers and their siblings. Nearly one third were described as having lots of friends, but 17% of the boys and 14% of the girls were described as having very few friends outside the immediate family. Two thirds of the sample had contact with friends outside school, but nearly one third of the children appeared to have no contact with school friends outside school hours. These findings suggest that there is a subgroup of children within the present sample, ranging from 15% to 33%, who appear to have very limited social relationships outside the immediate family.

Some 18% of the boys and 27% of the girls were suspected by their parents of persistently bullying other (usually younger) children. On the other hand 42% of the boys and 30% of the girls were themselves bullied by other children. Within the family 18% of the boys and 11% of the girls were reported as having poor or stormy relationships with their siblings. Twenty three percent of the boys and 25% of the girls showed no particular attachment to brothers or sisters in the family. Indeed 37% of disfluent boys and 25% of the girls were considered by their parents to be jealous of their own siblings. Here, the impression is of two groups of children, the smaller of the two being more aggressive towards other children whilst the larger group is more withdrawing and vulnerable in relation to their peers. Of course such behaviour does not occur in a vacuum and thus interviewers probe for the existence of current behavioural problems in the siblings of stuttering children in order to gauge the extent to which behaviour in disfluent children within the family is a reaction to the behaviour of their brothers and sisters. The reported rate of current behavioural problems in other siblings within the families of disfluent children was estimated at around 46% for male stutterers and 47% for female stutterers. Although a wide range of problems are subsumed within these proportions it appears that in many cases stuttering is only one of the problems that exist within the families of disfluent children, and this finding should influence the way in which treatment is formulated.

Child Development

Looking at individual **personality** and **temperament** traits parents were asked how their stuttering children adapt to meeting new people. Sixty percent of the boys and 50% of the girls were described as being hesitant and shy when confronted by new people, and a significant proportion of these children were also described as *'loners'*, even within the family circle. It would appear from this evidence that there is a significant subgroup of stuttering children who are considerably more withdrawn and less outgoing than the majority of children.

Family Position

The family position of stutterers in the sample is illustrated in Table 7. The distribution of birth

TABLE 7 Child Position in Family

SEX	Youngest	Middle	Eldest	Only Child
Boys	34%	10%	40%	16%
Girls	36%	7%	32%	25%

position clearly shows a bias in the sample towards youngest and eldest children. Even only children are represented to a greater degree in the sample than middle position children.

Relationships with Parents

Parents were asked to describe their usual relationship with the disfluent child. Well over three quarters of the children were said to have good relations with their mother, but a lower proportion had equally good relations with father. Interestingly, when asked who the child takes after 58% of the children were said to be like their fathers. When probing for particular emotional attachments to a parent it emerged that a fifth of the boys and nearly a third of the girls had a particular attachment to mother. For both boys and girls the proportion of children who had a particular attachment to father was only 7%. A further 28% of the boys and 37% of the girls had their special attachment to a specific grandparent, whilst 28% of boys and 16% of the girls had attachments to other adults outside the immediate family.

Clearly the rate of attachments to father is unexpectedly low in this sample, and this point is further emphasised by responses to the question *Who does the child confide in?* Three quarters of the boys and 92% of the girls were described as confiding exclusively in mother.

Only 10% of the boys confided in their father, and none of the girls in the sample were so described. Interestingly, when asked *which parent reprimands the child when he/she has been naughty?,* mothers emerged as the main disciplinarians for 30% of the boys and 50% of the girls. Fathers seldom reprimanded the children in this sample; only 9% of the boys and 5% of the girls were disciplined by father. Both parents were said to share responsibility for checking conduct in 61% of the boys and 45% of the girls.

Finally, a child's social and emotional behaviour is obviously influenced by the role models available within the family, and thus the interview technique probes for further indications of the **quality of parental relations**. Forty-two percent of the parents of male stutterers and 50% of the parents of female stutterers described their marital relationship as good. Some 10% of the parents of male stutterers and 22% of the parents of female stutterers indicated that their marital relationship was not completely satisfactory, with the atmosphere at home often being uncertain and volatile. The remaining proportion of parents did not offer a sufficiently convincing account of their marital relationship to classify it as either good or problematic. Our overall impression was that many of these parents did have significant relationship problems, but found it too difficult to discuss at such an early stage in the assessment and treatment process. If this was the case it would seem that a high proportion of the couples in this sample do not enjoy fulfilling relationships, and this may have consequences for children in such families.

Behaviour at School

Of particular significance for children in this age group is their attitude to school and their progress with formal education. In this sample a fairly high proportion of the children were attending private schools (31% of boys: 41% of girls). Parents claimed that most of the children enjoyed their school, though many indicated that unhappiness at previous schools had been the main reason for transfer from the state to the private sector. Roughly one third of the sample were reported to be making satisfactory progress at school according to their parents. Just over half the boys and 60% of the girls were described as making **average** progress, and 17% of the boys and 6% of the girls were experiencing marked academic difficulties at school. Whilst the only objective measure of school progress is the opinion of the child's teacher there can be little doubt that many children had been unsettled at school, and this had led to a high proportion of these children moving to new schools.

Child Development

Family History

During the parental interview an attempt is made to explore the wider family history in order to gain an understanding of the contribution of familial factors to childhood disfluency. This section begins with exploring details of mother's pregnancies, with particular attention to any difficulties surrounding the birth of the stuttering child. Twenty eight percent of the mothers reported a history of significant health difficulties during pregnancy and childbirth. Taking into account all pregnancies the main causes were miscarriages (83%), terminations (13%) and stillbirths (4%). Looking exclusively at the births of disfluent children in the 28% of mothers reporting complications some 71% of the mothers of male stutterers reported problems in the ante natal period as compared with 53% of the mothers of female stutterers. This is an unexpectedly high rate of complications amongst the disfluent children and warrants further detailed attention in future studies.

Turning to the developmental history of the parents themselves, a range of probes were used to elicit any specific difficulties, and this data is outlined in Table 8.

TABLE 8 Parental History

		MOTHER		FATHER	
BOYS	PROBLEM	Significant	Minimal	Significant	Minimal
	General Health	14%	13%	7%	15%
	Nervous Disorder	9%	8%	2%	7%
	Seen Psychiatrist	17%	-	3.5%	-
	Developmental/ Educational	5%	8%	6%	9%
	Emotional	11%	18%	3%	7%
	Stutter	12%	8%	21%	34%
GIRLS	General Health	7%	14%	11%	16%
	Nervous Disorder	4.5%	9%	9%	2%
	Seen Psychiatrist	7%	2%	14%	7%
	Developmental/ Educational	2%	11%	0	7%
	Emotional	16%	14%	9%	2%
	Stutter	11%	4%	32%	14%

15

Significant health problems were recorded in 14% of the mothers of male stutterers compared with 7% in female stutters. The rates were almost reversed amongst fathers. An unexpectedly high number of parents had consulted a psychiatrist for mental health problems at some point in their lives. Although the rates of significant nervous disorders are relatively low in the sample some 14% of the mothers of male stutterers and 14% of the fathers of female stutterers had sought professional advice for specific problems. Reports of emotional problems - typically bouts of anxiety and depression - were extremely common in this sample. Rates were significantly higher in mothers compared with fathers, but no clear sex differences emerged for the parents of stuttering boys and girls.

Rates of significant developmental/educational problems were relatively low, but in combination with problems judged by parents as minimal, there would appear to be a number of individuals with some history of educational and/or developmental difficulties. Finally, for both boys and girls the rate of disfluency amongst fathers is significantly higher than for mothers. This reflects known sex differences in the population.

Conclusion

This brief outline of the findings from the *childhood disfluency database* highlights the many problems that can exist in the families of stuttering children. No claim can be made for the representativeness of these findings, or their generalisation to other stuttering populations. However, it seems to us that even these broad findings do illustrate the need for a careful and systematic appraisal of the family dynamics as well as focusing on problems that child experiences in conjunction with disfluency. Many of the parents in our sample had experienced quite significant health and emotional problems during their lives, and a high proportion of the children clearly had multiple problems which extend beyond their disfluency. Whilst it may be tempting to view this evidence in terms of its etiological significance we would be more conservative in our interpretation. It seems enough simply to acknowledge that disfluency does not occur as an isolated problem in a child who exists in a vacuum. Understanding the contexts in which fluency problems arise, both in terms of the individual child and the family system in which that child is developing, offers considerable scope for more effective intervention.

The level of analysis reported here is deliberately descriptive; we have not attempted to report multi-dimensional profiles of subgroups of stuttering children, though this type of analysis is certainly possible. Rather, we have tried to convey some of the general findings from the childhood disfluency database which readers can explore for themselves. However, there appears to be two distinct extremes in child functioning within the present sample. As far as temperament and emotional behaviour is concerned it would seem there is a significant proportion of children who are consistently described by their parents as shy, withdrawing and socially isolated, often even within the family. These children are often bullied at school and have relatively few friends amongst their peers. At the other extreme lies a group of much more outgoing and adventurous children, who appear more likely to be bullies at school and who often require firm discipline from their parents. In the majority of these cases it is mother rather than father who acts as the chief disciplinarian. We have no doubt that the approach to treatment should differ for these subgroups. There may be other discernible subgroups of stutterers within the present sample who differ on other social and emotional dimensions. Here too, we would advocate that effective treatment for the individual case requires a careful analysis of the wider context in which disfluency occurs in order to address problems which may either be directly related, or at the very least may co-exist with disfluency.

Regardless of the specific therapeutic approach to the treatment of childhood disfluency it seems obvious that a detailed family interview procedure will generate valuable information which can be used to good effect during the treatment programme. Describing the social and emotional dynamics within families seems a good starting point for planning future parental involvement in the treatment process. In our experience the structured parental interview procedure yields many valuable insights into the workings of families and allows therapists to be sensitive to the history as well as the current problems being experienced by the family. This brief description of some of the key findings from the disfluency database may emphasise the value of the approach outlined here.

Parental Interview

Present Complaint

Detailed description of stuttering

How is the behaviour shown?

Date of onset?

Any major events at this time?

Frequency?   Severity?

Context: When is the stutter worst?

When is the stutter least?

What do you do when your child stutters?

Mother:

Father:

Other members of family:

How does the stutter affect the family?

Why are you seeking help now?

Recent behaviour and emotional state

General health

Away from school?   Stomach aches?

Asthma?   Sight?

Headaches?   Hearing?

Eating, sleeping and elimination

Eating difficulties at home or school?

Sleeping difficulties?

Nightmares?   Talking in sleep?

Sleepwalking?   Enuresis?   Soiling?

Regular bowel movement?

Muscular system and concentration

Overactive or restless?   Stay still if expected to?   Fidgety?

Concentration?   Longest time on something interesting?

Clumsiness?   Preferred hand and foot?

Speech

Speak as well as others of same age?   Difficulties in pronunciation?

Spontaneity of talking?

Tics and mannerisms

Twitches face or shoulders?

Blinking?   Nail-biting?

Sucking thumb?   Headbanging?

Soft toy or blanket?

3

Attack disorders

Faints?   Fits?   Petit Mal?

Emotions

Happy or miserable?   Crying?
Worried?

Irritable?

Temper?   Fears?   Sulking?
Tears on going to school?   School refusal?
Fussy?   Rituals?

Peer relationships

How does the child get on with other children?
Friends?   See them outside school?
Prefers children of own age?   Younger or older?
Girls or boys?   Leader or follower?
Bully?   Bullied?   Fights?
Teased?   Member of club?

Relationship with siblings

Position in the family?
Names and ages of siblings:
How do they get on?   How is this shown?
Particularly attached to any sibling?
Squabbling?   Who with?
Come to blows?   Jealousy?
Do the siblings have any particular problems?

Relationship with adults

How does the child get on with:
    mother?
    father?
Which child in the family do you relate to more easily?
    mother's reply:
    father's reply:
How does the child compare with other children?
How is affection shown?
Is the child easy to get on with?   Who does the child take after?
In what ways does the child get on your nerves?
    mother's reply:
    father's reply:
How does the child get on with other adults?   With teachers?

4

Anti-social trends

Disobedient?

Fire setting?

Stealing?

   At home or outside?

Truanting?

Smoke?

Drugs?

Destructive?

Lies?

On own or with others?

Run away?

Drinks?

Trouble with police?

Sex education

Interest in opposite sex?

Instructed in sex?

Masturbation?

Questions asked?

Menstruation?

Schooling

Which school/s attended (including nursery placement)?

Like it?

Progress: Reading?

        Writing?

           Other?

Reports?

Do parents see the teacher?

Family structure and history

How long married/together?

Previous marriages/children?

Previous long-term relationships/children?

Mother's pregnancies, abortions, miscarriages or still births?

Children adopted or fostered?

Number in home?

Personal background	Mother	Father
Place of birth		
Age		
Religion		
Occupation		
Education		
General health/illness		

Personal background	Mother	Father
Description of personality		
Depression?		
Seen by psychiatrist?		
Difficulty learning to read or speak		
Emotional problems		
Stuttering (any treatment?)		
Left-handed		
Enuretic		
Alcoholism		
Epilepsy		
Court appearances		

Parents' family background	Mother	Father
Siblings		
Upbringing		

The child's grandparents	Maternal grandparents	Paternal grandparents
Occupation		
Current contact		
(Date and cause of death)		

Extended family issues	Mother's family	Father's family
Psychiatric treatment		
Depression		
Suicide/attempt		
Slow to speak		
Stuttering		
Difficulty learning to read		
Left handed		
Enuretic		
Mental illness		
Alcoholism		
Epilepsy		
Court appearances		

21

6

Home circumstances

House or flat?

Sleeping arrangements?

Number of bedrooms?

Others in home?

Finances

Any difficulties?

Neighbourhood

How long lived there?

Do you like it?

Family life and relationships

Parental relationships

How do you get on?

Things enjoyed doing together?

How spend evenings and weekends?

Father's participation in child care and household tasks?

How would the child's life be different is he did not stutter?

How do parents resolve problems in the family?

Parent-child interaction

Activities child enjoys?

Go out together?

Play together?

Help with homework?

Help make things?

Child's participation in family activities

Help with dressing?   Feeding?

Who helps?

Taken to school?

Does the child help with washing up, shopping, errands, etc?

Family relationships

Is the child a 'mother's child' or a 'father's child'?

Confide in father?

mother?

Attachment to other adults?

Discipline

Bedtime regulations (including time?)

Allowed to climb on furniture?

Allowed to leave house without saying where going?

Restrictions on friends: Reading: TV:

Who reprimands?

What method of punishment is used?

Pocket money?

Amount:

Child's developmental history

Pregnancy
Mother's health during pregnancy?
Home or hospital delivery?
Maturity?   Birthweight?
Health after pregnancy?

Neonatal period
Difficulties breathing or sucking?
Convulsions?   Jaundice?

Feeding
Breast or bottle?   Weaning when?   Introduction of solids?

Development in infancy
Placid or active?   Crying?   Response to mother?

Milestones
Sitting unsupported?   Walking?
First words with meaning?   First three-word phrases?
Comparison with siblings?
Any developmental problems?

Bladder and bowel control
When obtained?
Day: Night: Problems:

Illnesses
Ever been in hospital? In patient:
                    Outpatient:
Clinic: (a) Speech
        (b) Child guidance
        (c) Other, including accident and emergency
Serious illnesses?

Separations
Ever away from home without parents?
Apart from parents (holidays, hospitals, etc)
How looked after?
Reaction?

Other comments

8

Temperamental or personality attributes

Meeting new people

Adults?   Children?

Go up to strangers?

Shy or clinging?   How quickly does the child adapt to someone new?

New situations

Reaction to: (a) New places: does the child explore or hang back?

(b) New gadgets?

(c) New foods?

How quick to adapt?

Emotional expression

How vigorous in expression of feelings?

Sensitivity

How does the child respond if a person or an animal is hurt?

How does the child react if something goes wrong?

Additional comments

Note rate of parents' speech

Note future impending changes

How do parents resolve problems in the family?

Summary of issues

Management

Chapter 2

Young Stutterers' Speech Production: Some Clinical Implications

Edward G. Conture & Ellen M. Kelly

The purpose of this chapter is to discuss recent research regarding young stutterers' speech production and some implications this has for the clinical management of childhood stuttering. These research findings have tremendous potential for influencing the clinician's thinking about and planning for the clinical diagnosis and remediation of young stutterers. To provide some context for how these findings may be of clinical benefit, we will start by briefly reviewing recent history in the area of stuttering theory and therapy.

Some Brief History

From the end of World War II to about 1970, the pendulum of interest in stuttering had swung far from the **nature** (i.e. constitutional, genetic, organic or physiological influences) to the **nurture** (i.e. environmental, psychological or social influences) side of the continuum. Representative of, as well as influential in this period, were such approaches as Johnson's diagnosogenic theory (e.g. Johnson and Associates 1959), various learning theory formulations (cf. Bloodstein 1987), and the psychodynamics of Sheehan's (1958, 1975) conflict or double approach-avoidance theories. In essence, during this period environmental, learning, psychological, and social issues held most of the attention.

In the late 1960's and early 1970's, however, several events coincided to send the pendulum swinging back in the direction of nature including: (1) the emergence of speech science as a discipline, with its exacting methodologies and rich but hotly contested theories regarding the nature of human speech communication, (2) Wingate's (1969, 1970) speculations that the *distraction hypothesis* (cf. Bloodstein 1987) inadequately explains why stutterers become fluent when speaking in the presence of high-level noise and rhythmic stimulation (cf. Beech & Fransella 1968), (3) Van Riper's (1971) speculation that stuttering relates to a temporal discoordination among the respiratory, phonatory and articulatory systems, and (4) Schwartz's (1974) speculation that laryngeal disruptions may *cause* instances of stuttering. Shortly thereafter, researchers and clinicians alike turned their attention back to the nature side of the continuum, and focused on genetic (e.g. Kidd 1983) and physiological (e.g. Adams *et al* 1984) parameters to try and better understand the problem of stuttering.

In the mid 1970's through early 1980's most work centered on studies of stutterers' laryngeal behavior and their voice onset and reaction times (cf. Adams *et al* 1984; Starkweather 1982). In the 1980's, researchers began to directly study the speech production skills of stutterers; particularly those of adults who stutter. Discussion ensued regarding: (1) whether or not such investigations should focus on stutterers' stuttered or fluent utterances, (2) whether disturbances are mainly temporal, spatial or both (e.g. Caruso, Abbs & Gracco 1988) and (3) whether or not one could readily extrapolate from findings with adults who stutter and apply them to children who stutter and vice versa (e.g. Conture 1987). Most of this work, as noted above, involved adults who stutter and for reasons to be discussed below, we believed that the speech production abilities and behavior of children who stutter also needed to be studied.

Young Stutterers' Speech Production: Results of Syracuse Project

From the late 1970's to present, the first author, his colleagues and doctoral students have been studying the speech production and related behavior of children who stutter (e.g. Conture *et al* 1986, 1988; Zebrowski & Conture 1989). It is not the purpose of this chapter to review each and every one of these papers or associated clinical writings regarding youngsters who stutter (e.g. Conture & Fraser 1989; Conture 1990b) or the related studies of others. Instead, we would like to relate some of our research findings regarding these young children to the clinical process.

We initially set out to assess the *temporal discoordination* hypothesis (cf. Van Riper 1971) and related speculation regarding the stuttered and fluent speech of children who stutter. In essence, this hypothesis suggests that stuttering relates to a temporal breakdown or disruption in the complex interactions and coordinations between respiratory, phonatory and articulatory events needed to produce speech. We had no *a priori* notion that these temporal disruptions resulted from central (e.g. cortical) and/or peripheral (e.g. lower motor neurons) sources. Neither did we know in advance whether these temporal disruptions, if they existed, were even observable to the instrumentally-unaided eye or ear. We simply reasoned that if they contribute to stuttering, they should somehow be manifest in the speech of young stutterers.

The assumption that children are not small adults. We studied preschool and early elementary school-age youngsters who stutter because we thought this would increase the likelihood that any observed aberrations in speech production were not the result of the *well-established, long-term history of stuttering* typical of that exhibited by adults who stutter. We also thought that *...such youngsters have had less time than adult stutterers to develop reactions to stuttering and speech in general. Such reactions would contaminate, for the purposes of investigation, observations of speech production behavior* (Conture *et al* 1988: p. 641). We assumed that *...the temporal parameters of coordination associated with young stutterers' stutterings are less likely to be "contaminated" by compensatory/coping reactions than those of adult stutterers* (Caruso *et al* 1988: p. 59). In essence, since children go through a myriad of changes (e.g. social, emotional, linguistic, cognitive, motoric, etc.) as they develop, we reasoned that it would be problematic to assume that a child who stutters would be similar to an adult who stutters in terms of their speech production abilities and behavior. It is quite possible that there are important differences between children and adults who stutter may in terms of the origin, course and/or symptomatology of their problem. Increasing our understanding of these differences should help us develop clinical procedures that are better suited to meet the special needs and concerns of children versus adults who stutter.

Young stutterers' fluent speech. We were primarily interested in studying young stutterers' perceptibly *fluent* speech since we wanted to know if these children exhibit disruptions in speech production throughout the entirety of their speech (i.e. the fluent as well as disfluent aspects). Possibly, disruptions noted associated with stuttering, as Conture *et al* (1986: p. 384) suggested, might be *...exacerbated versions or more elaborate versions of aberrations associated with their perceptually fluent speech.* Although finding temporal disruptions during young stutterers' stutterings would be revealing, we thought that it would be unclear whether *...these disruptions are merely reactions to some other aspect of the stuttering act* (Conture *et al* 1986: p. 384) or whether they contribute to the instance of stuttering. Therefore, we studied both the fluent as well as stuttered aspects of young stutterers' speech.

In our first published study (Zebrowski *et al* 1985) we reported no significant mean difference between young stutterers and their normally fluent peers on a variety of temporal acoustic measures of the perceptually fluent productions of /p/ and /b/, a finding consistent with that of Pindzola (1986) with adult stutterers. Interestingly, however, Zebrowski *et al* (1985) reported a negative correlation (r = -0.41) between normally fluent youngsters' aspiration duration and stop gap duration but no such relation for young stutterers (r = 0.14), a finding somewhat similar to that of Borden *et al* 1987) with adult stutterers. Aspiration duration, usually measured in milliseconds (ms), refers to the duration of weak, diffuse acoustic energy associated with vocal-fold approximation that occurs, for example, in the word *pea*, between the ending of supra-glottal release of the /p/ and the beginning of voicing for the /i/. Stop gap duration (in ms) refers to the duration of absent or minimal acoustic energy that occurs, for example, during the phrase *see pete*, between the ending of acoustic energy of the /i/ in *see* and the beginning of acoustic energy associated with the supra-glottal release for the /p/ in *pete*.These apparently subtle disruptions in young stutterers' temporal *trading relations* between supraglottal (e.g. stop-gap) and laryngeal (e.g. aspiration) events were taken to suggest that the entirety of young stutterers' speech production, not just their stutterings, is subtly atypical. Perhaps, these subtle disruptions in speech production, may represent a less efficient means of producing speech and one that is more sensitive to being further disrupted by untoward environmental stressors.

Conture *et al* (1986) provided further evidence that young stutterers' fluent speech may contain brief, subtle disruptions. They reported that during consonant-vowel (CV) or vowel-consonant (VC), normally fluent children exhibited significantly more *typical* (72% of total measured CV/VC transitions) vocal fold abduction patterns than did children who stutter (42% of total measured CV/VC transitions). It was speculated that *...some young stutterers tend to have difficulty stabilizing and controlling laryngeal gestures even during speech judged fluent by trained listeners, particularly at those points in the utterance where these youngsters must move between sound segments* (Conture *et al* 1986: p. 384).

In contrast, to the above studies which employed relatively short duration, subtle measures of young stutterers' speech production, Conture *et al* (1988) employed fairly gross temporal measures of young stutterers' speech production (e.g. onset of respiratory deflation [i.e. beginning of exhalation] relative to the onset of lower lip opening). Using these relatively gross temporal measures to study temporal relations between and within young stutterers' respiratory, phonatory and articulatory behavior, Conture *et al* (1988) reported neither statistically significant nor apparent differences between the perceptually fluent speech of young stutterers and that of their normally fluent peers in terms of selected temporal measures of speech production, a finding consistent with Schwartz (1987) who studied another group of young stutterers. It was concluded that the gross *...temporal characteristics of coordination for young stutterers' fluent speech production(s) are not appreciably different from those of their normally fluent peers and further, any temporal characteristics of stutterers' fluent speech that do differ from normal are probably brief, as well as subtle, in nature* (Conture *et al* 1988: p. 640).

Thus, the perceptibly fluent speech of children who stutter seems to contain, at the most, relatively brief, subtle, rather than long, grossly apparent, disruptions in speech production. As we will discuss below, however, it is entirely possible, however, that these brief, subtle *temporal asynchronies* in young stutterers' perceptibly fluent speech may be sufficient, if not necessary, to put these children **at risk** for developing stuttering. Indeed, these slight temporal asynchronies may be compounded or exacerbated by the untoward influences of internal (e.g. the need to quickly formulate a complex answer to a question) as well as external (e.g. a listeners consistent tendency to rush and interrupt the child) environmental stressors.

Young stutterers' stuttered speech. While our main thrust was to determine whether the entirety, not just the stuttered aspects, of young stutterers' speech was temporally disturbed, we did complete two studies of young stutterers' stutterings (Caruso *et al* 1988; Schwartz 1987). Caruso *et al* (1988) found, however, that the sequences of temporal coordination both **within** a particular component of the speech production system (e.g. supraglottal articulation) and **between** different components (e.g. supraglottal articulation and phonation) were not significantly different between normally fluent children and the stuttered utterances of their stuttering peers. Although Caruso *et al* (1988) reported that the absolute mean onsets of young stutterers' various speech production events were typically earlier - thus being longer in duration - *...the relative temporal sequence of these same events during stutterings was comparable to that associated with normally fluent children's fluent productions* (p. 57).

Related to this study was Schwartz and Conture's (1988) finding of 5 significantly different subgroups of young stutterers based on speech and nonspeech behavior associated with instances of stuttering. Schwartz (1987) also assessed whether these *behavioral* subgroups are correlated with *physiological* subgroups, using essentially the same physiological measures reported by Caruso *et al* (1988). While Schwartz (1987) sampled less than the 43 young stutterers used by Schwartz and Conture, his study of 10 randomly selected stutterings produced by each of 15 randomly selected young stutterers from these 43 indicated that there were no significant difference in temporal coordinations during stutterings across the various subgroups. Schwartz's findings suggests that significant behavioral differences between young stutterers are not associated with significant differences in speech production between these children, at least for the relatively gross measures of temporal coordination in speech that were employed.

Summary of Syracuse project: Subtle differences between stutterers and their normally fluent peers. Our various studies of young stutterers' speech production all seem to support the same conclusion: no significant differences were found between the perceptibly fluent speech of young stutterers and that of normally fluent youngsters in terms of relatively gross, temporal measures of respiratory, phonatory or articulatory behavior. However, it should immediately be cautioned that finding no significant differences does not mean that the two groups are identical or exactly alike in terms of their speech production. Non-significant differences simply mean that differences we observed were not appreciably different from those we might expect to find by chance alone by sampling any two groups of children. For example, normally fluent youngsters' average onset time for lip closing for word-initial bilabial sounds (/p b f v m w/) occurred non-significantly sooner than that of children who stutter (Conture *et al* 1988).

Some important caveats. Regardless of future methodological refinements, it is and will remain extremely difficult to discriminate between disruptions in speech production that **cause** versus those which are **symptoms** of versus those which are **reactions** to instances of stuttering. No one, it would seem, can claim that a behavior that is **part** of an instance of stuttering can also **cause** or **precipitate** the same instance of stuttering. Likewise, no one can presently claim to know the speed or duration of a young child's **reactions** to his or her own speech behavior and whether the brief, subtle aberrations in young stutterers' speech production can be meaningfully considered as a child's *reaction* to his or her own speech behavior. Perhaps, as Williams (1957) suggested, stuttering is a process that begins prior to and continues after the instance of overt stuttering. Thus, disruptions observed during the perceptibly fluent speech of young stutterers may represent: (1) a *spreading* of disruptions

30

in young stutterers' speech production into adjacent speech segments, (2) speech production manifestations of young stutterers' anticipations of stuttering on future words, or (3) young stutterers' overall hesitant, tentative manner of speech production. Likewise, we still don't know whether the brief, subtle disturbances we observed during young stutterers' perceptibly fluent speech differ in **kind** (i.e. different types) versus **degree** (i.e. different frequencies of occurrence) from those disruptions observed during their instances of stuttering.

There is also no evidence that the brief, subtle disruptions in speech production exhibited by young stutterers were **never** exhibited by normally fluent children. Instead, it should be pointed out, these disruptions were exhibited **more frequently** by young stutterers than by normally fluent children. Similarly to numerical differences in speech disfluencies between normally fluent and stuttering children, the two talker groups differ numerically (i.e., in terms of the **frequency of occurrence** of their behavior) rather than categorically (i.e. in terms of the **nature** of their behavior) in terms of aberrations in their speech production. Simply put, children who stutter produce more of the same behaviors than their normally fluent peers produce, at least during their perceptibly fluent utterances. It will require some time and a good deal of research to determine whether disruptions in speech production associated with the stuttered or fluent speech of children or adults who stutter are (1) symptoms (2) reactions or (3) initiators of stuttering or some complex mix of 2 or more of these possibilities.

Young Stutterers' Speech Production: Alternative Routes Hypothesis

Many routes to the same destination. One interpretation of the above findings is that there are many possible speech production routes that lead to the same end (i.e. reasonably intelligible, fluent speech) and that certain routes are probably used most often by most speakers. However, one *alternative* route, seemingly used more often by young stutterers than their normally fluent peers, appears to be characterized by **more** inefficient means of moving from sound to sound or of initiating sounds. This alternative route will lead to the same end but do so by sacrificing the speed, precision, rhythm or forward flow of speech production. The number and nature of alternative routes that children may use to achieve fluent speech is unclear, but it is likely that some are more stable than others and more resistant to the untoward influences of external (i.e. listener) as well as internal (i.e. speaker) environmental stressors.

Alternative, inefficient routes may be less resistant to environmental stressors. We have speculated elsewhere (Conture 1990b) that some routes are much more resistant than others to **environmental stressors**; for example, interruptions of the child by listeners, listeners who require or encourage the child to use rapid, mature and precise speech, listeners' verbal or nonverbal messages that they don't like the manner and content of the child's speech, listeners' verbal or nonverbal indications that they are not paying attention to the child, and so forth. If a child is frequently exposed to these environmental stressors **and** he or she tends to use, for whatever reason, an alternative route to produce speech, the child may be at risk for stuttering. This combination of environmental stressors **plus** alternative routes of speech production may explain why some children, who are frequently exposed to environmental stressors but use a more typical manner of speech production, experience very little if any speech disfluencies. Whether, on the other, these inefficient types of speech production are sufficient to lead to stuttering, in the absence of environmental stressors, is a question that must await future research.

We believe that this tendency towards using more inefficient methods of speech production is probably not something the child learns to do but is something that is an integral aspect of his or her developing speech production system. For some of these youngsters, these inefficiencies in speech production are probably of minimal consequence and will decrease as the child grows older. With other youngsters, however, these inefficiencies remain throughout much of childhood (and beyond), keeping them at risk for developing and maintaining stuttering. For example, we may hypothesize that those children who exhibit articulation/phonological problems along with stuttering (cf. Louko *et al* in press) may tend to produce more of these inefficiencies than young stutterers who don't exhibit phonological problems. This, however, is an empirical question that must await further research for an answer.

The point for clinicians here is that there are probably many different speech production routes to the same end: perceptibly fluent speech. While some routes might be maximally resistant to environmental stressors - for example, listeners interruptions of and demands that the child speed up speech production - other speech production routes might be less resistant. Perhaps many children who stutter produce the entirety of their speech in ways that make them much more susceptible than the typical child to the everyday slings and arrows of external and internal stressors that all children experience. To paraphrase what we have said elsewhere (Conture 1990b), we think that stuttering relates to a complex interaction between the child's environment (which in this case may be exposing the child to a wide variety and high frequency of stressors) and the skills and abilities the child brings to that environment (which in this case may be a tendency to consistently produce speech in a subtly inefficient manner).

Young Stutterers' Speech Production: Some Intellectual Influences On Clinicians

How should we measure a child's speech fluency? Traditionally, speech disfluency has been perceptually measured by listeners who, with training, can arrive at a reasonable degree of intra-judge and inter-judge reliability at least in terms of overall frequency of occurrence (cf. Conture 1990a; Young 1984). Traditionally, speech production (i.e. the complex of temporal and spatial acts and coordinations of respiratory, phonatory and articulatory behaviors) has been objectively measured through the use of various forms of instrumentation. Speech production is that event which creates the acoustic signal that listeners perceive, in whole or in part. It is this perception of the acoustic signal, then, that is evaluated or judged as being fluent or disfluent. Therefore, researchers' descriptions of their instrumentally-aided observations of speech production will probably differ from listeners' descriptions of their perceptual observations of the resulting acoustic speech signal. This is so because researchers using instrumentation and observers using their own perceptual judgments are observing different aspects of the same speech utterances and rely on different observational procedures to arrive at their descriptions and judgments. Furthermore, research findings make it clear (e.g. Atal *et al* 1978) that the relation between speech acoustics and speech production is anything but a simple, one-to-one relationship. Whatever the case, some might ask whether observers would perceive an individual as producing fluent speech even though that individual is exhibiting speech that may be described as physiologically disfluent?

Perceptual versus instrumentally-aided observations. Answering the preceding question essentially boils down to making a distinction between **overt** (i.e. discernable to the instrumentally-unaided eye or ear) versus **covert** (i.e. discernable only instrumentally) indications of disfluency. Must we assume that speech production is only *correct, normal or typical,* if it contains absolutely NO physiological disruptions (i.e. is physiologically ideal or perfect)? This would seem to be a bit like assuming that our manner of walking is only physiologically normal or correct if we **never** slip, stumble, trip, or turn our ankle. This neither suggests that physiological disruptions are unimportant to typical speech production nor that they are unrelated to the initiation, maintenance or exacerbation of stuttering.

What it does suggest is that it may be inappropriate to use the term *fluent* or *disfluent* when describing aberrations, disruptions or disturbances in speech production that are not correlated with or do not result in an instrumentally-unaided listener judgments of speech disfluency. Instead, it would appear to be less confusing to reserve the use of these terms for the description of our perceptual observations of the acoustic signal and/or associated speech production and use such terms as *aberrations, disruptions, disturbances, discoordinations, asynchronies* and so forth, when describing instrumentally-detected departures from *typical* speech production. To draw an analogy, we may be able to make gross perceptual distinctions between cold and hot in terms of room temperature but are probably less able to perceive changes in room temperature of 1 or 2 degrees on the thermometer. Likewise, we may be able to make relatively gross perceptual distinctions between fluent and disfluent speech but we are probably less able to perceive changes in speech production of one or two milliseconds. Of course, the real issue is not whether listeners' observations differ from instrumentally-aided observations of young stutterers' speech, but which of these two forms of observations is most useful to us in furthering our understanding, diagnosis and treatment of stuttering. Suffice it to say, that resolution of this issue will require a great deal of thought and effort on the parts of clinicians and researchers alike.

Can clinicians perceive brief, subtle disruptions with the naked eye and ear? The preceding discussion strongly suggests that we don't know the answer to this question. It is our experience that most of these behaviors are imperceptible to all but the most highly trained observer. This shouldn't lead us to disregard these behaviors any more than a doctor would disregard micro-organisms simply because the doctor needed a microscope or laboratory tests to observe the micro-organisms. Evidence of these inefficiencies may include slightly inappropriate: supra-glottal articulation, pauses within or between sounds or syllables and/or onset, offset or quality (i.e. breathy, hoarse, etc.) of voicing and other such events.

What we may find, with further experimental and clinical research, is that certain instrumental procedures, for example the electroglottograph, quite accurately and reliably record disruptions in speech production that listeners judge to be fluent. It is unknown whether these short duration, relatively subtle disruptions in speech production change during speech therapy. If they do change during therapy, and such changes are related to long-term improvement, clinicians will need to know more about using and interpreting such instrumentation in order to augment their assessment of therapeutic progress (cf. Colton & Conture, 1990 for review of research and clinical use of the electroglottograph). Maybe those young stutterers for whom such inefficiencies do not change during therapy are those children who continue to stutter into adulthood. Once again, these are empirical issues that can only be answered through further clinically-oriented research.

What is the nature of the speech production of young stutterers' during stutterings?. We found, much to our surprise, that the temporal sequences of onsets during young stutterers' instances of stuttering were not significantly different than those during comparable fluent utterances produced by normally fluent children. These findings might be taken to suggest that young stutterers are able to control at least the temporal aspects of speech and/or voice initiation, but it is their apparent inability to complete or move on to the next sound that makes them repeat and prolong speech sounds and syllables. In other words, young stutterers have more difficulties with the **offset** (linking or transitional behavior) than the **onset** (initiating or starting aspects) of speech production! Certainly, our findings provide little support for the notion that inappropriate onset that keep the stutterer from making the proper subsequent transitional movement (this would be like, as Van Riper [1971] suggested, hitting the wrong first key on a piano when trying to play a musical piece).

Chasing the "cause" from one organ to another. Our seemingly constant search for the single flaw that accounts for the complex problem of stuttering appears to be part of the problem rather than the solution. It will be recalled that some (e.g. Orton & Travis 1929; Travis & Knott 1936, 1937) have speculated that stuttering is caused by cortical dysfunction while others have speculated that laryngeal problems cause stuttering (e.g. Schwartz 1974). This one problem - one organ mentality (e.g. problem: stuttering - organ: brain) on the part of both researchers and clinicians has seemingly caused us to search from one site to the next in hopes of finding the place where stuttering originates. It is as we have been chasing stuttering from one organ to another! Like those trying to pin the cause of crime on one factor (e.g. drugs), we continually scrutinize the stutterer and his or her environment for the **one** factor that causes stuttering. Our experience to date should tell us, however, that stuttering, like crime, relates to an interaction among **variety** of issues. Thus, no single variable can adequately account for stuttering (or crime, for that matter).

Related to the unidimensional-solutions-to-multidimensional-problems issue, is the notion that there is a fixed or stationary problem that accounts for the highly variable behavior called stuttering. Young stutterers, according to some of our data, may have less than precise control over certain aspects of their speech production mechanism, findings which might be taken to suggest that disruptions in speech production or underlying neuromotor control causes stuttering. However, if disruptions in the neuromotor *control* for speech production cause children to stutter, such difficulties must be variable in nature since young stutterers not infrequently stutter on a sound in the first part of an utterance that they produce fluently later in the utterance. Particularly in children, stuttering waxes and wanes between and within days, weeks and months. Those who believe that difficulties in neuromotor control cause stuttering need to consider why these difficulties may be manifest in certain speaking situations (e.g. talking to an inattentive listener) but not in others (e.g. talking to a younger sibling about shared toys). Serious thought must be given to how a constant neuromotor problem readily and totally accounts for the highly variable nature of stuttering that is the hallmark of childhood stuttering

Young Stutterers' Speech Production: Some Practical Implications For Clinicians

Neuromotor testing. Perhaps young stutterers' brief, subtle disruptions in speech production are somehow related to delays and/or deviations in one or more aspects of these youngsters' neuromotor development for speech. This suggests that speech-language pathologists will probably want to refine and/or improve their abilities to screen for neuromotor development relative to speech. Unfortunately, as any clinician who has tried to assess the neuromotor abilities of children under 7 years of age can tell us, wanting to test the neuromotor skills of young children is one thing while actually doing so is an entirely different matter! Many of these young children fatigue quickly as soon as they give their undivided attention to such tasks as alternating motion rate (i.e. diadochokinesis). These youngsters also vary a great deal in terms of their abilities to understand and follow test instructions. Most importantly, however, children under 7 years of age exhibit a great deal of normal variation within and between themselves in terms of oral and non-oral neuromotor skills. Even when employing published guidelines for the neurological examination of children (e.g. Peters *et al* 1975), we must ever be open to the idea that young stutterers have just as much right as normally fluent children to have problems with their neuromotor development. Thus, a co-occurrence of stuttering and delays in neuromotor development does not necessarily mean that one causes the other.

In our opinion, Fletcher's (1972) time-by-count method for scoring alternating motion rate or diadochokinetic syllable rates (i.e. the client is asked to repeat uni-, bi- or tri-syllables with the clinician counting the first ten production and timing the length of time needed to say the 10) is the best way to assess diadochokinesis in children under 7 years of age. Clinicians should be cautioned, particularly when studying young stutterers' alternating motion rates for uni-, bi- or tri-syllables, to exclude from their counts any syllables where an overt stuttering is apparent. If a clinician includes instances of stutterings or stuttering-like behavior in the results of diadochokinetic testing, such inclusion will not only significantly influence the number of syllables counted but also the length of time it takes the child to produce ten syllables.

Riley & Riley (1985) published the *Oral Motor Assessment Scale* to assess ...*correct voicing, smooth coarticulation, proper sequencing and age appropriate rate of syllable* and they believe that such testing will help detect *oral motor discoordination* in children. Many clinicians and researchers appear to believe that a sizable number of children who stutter also exhibit oral motor discoordination, but until recently there was limited data with which to evaluate such speculation. Recently, Byrd & Cooper (1989) used the *Screening Test for Developmental Apraxia of Speech* (STDAS; Blakeley 1980) to study apraxic, stuttering and normally fluent children. There were significant differences in mean overall STDAS scores between the three talker groups. But when differences between the three talker groups were examined for each of the eight STDAS subtests, only the articulation subtest scores for the young stutterers were significantly different from those of children labelled as *apraxic* and only the expressive language discrepancy and prosody subtests for the young stutterers significantly differed from that of those of the normally fluent children. Thus, there is some behavioral evidence that children who stutter seem to differ from normally fluent children in terms of overall neuromotor development; however, it is unknown what the underlying reasons for these differences are and whether they make a difference in terms of stuttering in children.

Of course, unless clinicians actually test for and find delays and/or deviations with young stutterers neuromotor development, they should not assume a priori that young stutterers have such problems. Besides, even if a child does exhibit such difficulties, there is nothing to indicate that the underlying reasons for these difficulties are immutable to environmental influences nor impervious to the effects of development and/or therapy. These children can and should be helped but the form and length of such helping may need to be tailored to these youngsters' special needs.

Holding one's breath. For the clinician who doesn't stutter, it is difficult to get a physical as well as emotional feeling of what it is like to stutter. This problem is one of the reasons that training programs have, for years, sent students out into everyday society to stutter on purpose. This practice, however, does not tell the clinician how stuttering **physically feels** for any one particular stutterer. Certainly, it is important that clinicians are able to quickly and accurately hear instances of stuttering, but hearing is only part of what the stutterer senses. The stutterer also physically feels instances of stuttering. Thus, to gain a better appreciation of what the stutterer senses during stuttering, it is instructive to have clients who stutter do the following two manoeuvres:

(1) Take a deep breath and hold it with your mouth open.

(2) Take a deep breath and hold it with your lips closed and your cheeks puffed out.

After each of these manoeuvres, the clinician can ask the client *is that what it feels like when you stutter?* The clinician might even ask the client to push with the respiratory system or may even place a hand on the client's stomach and push in. Clients who primarily *lock* at the level of larynx will say that it feels like (1) above, while those who primarily fixate at the level of the mouth will associate (2) above. Some clients will mention that it feels like both (1) and (2). This is a good procedure for helping the stutterer understand that **some** of the pressure or tension they feel in the area of their neck and/or throat is a build-up of air pressure resulting from the egressive air flow from their lungs being impeded by laryngeal and/or supralaryngeal closure. Having this information should help the client understand that these feelings are not the result of a sound, syllable or word *caught* or *stuck* in their throat, lungs or stomach.

Summary and Conclusions

In the past twenty years, we have begun to accumulate some information about the temporal and spatial aspects of speech production associated with the perceptibly fluent speech of young stutterers. At this point, it appears that there are no gross temporal or spatial aberrations in the perceptibly fluent speech of young stutterers but some brief, subtle aberrations in speech production have been reported. It is unclear whether these brief, subtle disruptions in young stutterers perceptibly fluent speech are different in degree or kind from those that they may exhibit during stuttering. The answer to this question will take a series of studies with a variety of young subjects to clarify. This sort of information lends some support to the current clinical *zeitgeist* whereby stuttering is treated as if it involved a disruption in the temporal and/or spatial aspects of speech production (i.e. disruptions in *time and tension*; Conture 1990b).

The influence of the above information on clinicians is primarily, at this point, intellectual. By this we mean that such information may be used to expand clinicians' information base, provide them with different perspectives and help with the planning of when and for whom therapy should begin. These intellectual influences have real potential for clinical practice, but researchers don't set out to tell clinicians **how to** do therapy anymore than clinicians set out to tell researchers **how to** conduct their research. Researchers and clinicians are involved in complimentary endeavors. Researchers function primarily to expand and improve the knowledge base (i.e. *to seek the truth*), while clinicians work to apply this knowledge to the clinical management of stuttering. Having both groups share ideas with one another and keep abreast of trends in each other's areas of endeavor increases the chances that their related but different activities will lead to a better understanding of stuttering and improvement in the clinical diagnosis as well as management of this problem.

Acknowledgment. This chapter was made possible in part by a NINCDS contract (NO1-NS-0-2331) and OSEP grants (GO000850252 and HO23C8OO8) to Syracuse University.

Chapter 3

Interactions With Pre-Operational Pre-School Stutterers: How Will This Influence Therapy?

Susan C. Meyers

What is Known and Unknown About Interaction?

Previous stuttering research has focused on the theory that the parents' interactions shape the development, persistence, and maintenance of a child's stutter. This early research into parent-child interaction was **unidirectional** in that the parent's behaviour was the only focus. As a result of this limited focus, counselling to remediate the parent's negative interactional patterns was the preferred method of treatment for the family of a preschool stutterer (see Chapter 4 for discussion).

Counselling generated from unidirectional thinking was based on one of two premises. The first was general to all parent-child relationships and overall communication while the second premise was specific to stuttering. From a global perspective, improvement of parenting skills (of discipline, feeding, and bedtime routines) and other positive modifications of the home and family environment was considered helpful for any child, and may have been especially important for children with problems. If this generalized improvement in the child's home-life was in fact needed and was the basis for altering the parental interactions, then counselling was most likely justified.

The second and more direct premise called for modification of parental patterns of verbal interaction to reduce the child's frequency of stuttering. For example, parents were counselled to speak more slowly and to reduce the number of open-ended questions, interruptions, negative comments, criticisms and inappropriate vocabulary (Ainsworth 1988; Gregory & Hill 1984; Riley & Riley 1983).

Unidirectional research was experientially-based on clinical intuitiveness (Perkins 1980). It has been difficult to determine from reviewing stuttering research on parent counselling whether or not a child's improvement in fluency was solely due to the modification(s) of the parental verbal interaction. It is possible that children considered *stutterers* a) were not really stutterers but normally disfluent speakers, b) regained fluency because they had received direct intervention from a speech-language pathologist, or c) improved because of motoric and linguistic maturation. As Quarrington (1966) suggested, the verbal relationship between the parent and stutterer may be the key factor in the etiology of stuttering. In other words, the development, persistence, and maintenance of stuttering is a **bidirectional** process involving both the listener and stutterer. The interpretation of current research adds support to this bidirectional model.

More recently, research in child development has operated from a bidirectional perspective. The premise is that the child contributes to the interactive relationship as much as does the parent. Development is then defined as a dynamic process of interlocking reactions between the child and others in the child's environment (Kuo 1976). Thus, a child has its own repertoire of prior environmental experiences. Effects on social behaviour can be biological in nature, neurologically predetermined, or directly influenced in relationship to interacting with others in the environment. Variables such as contact with the mother and father, quantitative time within the partner-child relationship, temperament of the child, and verbal experiences offered in the environment may be the essential factors involved in the communicative development of a child. Current research endeavors focus on the verbal interactions of the child as well as the parent. This bidirectional theory may explain why one child has the predisposition to stutter and a sibling within the same family maintains fluency.

To investigate the possibility that stuttering may be influenced by the bidirectional relationship (between a stutterer and a partner), Meyers and Freeman (1985a,b,c) cross-matched mothers (of stutterers and nonstutterers) interacting with their own and other preschool children. Interpretation of findings were that all mothers interrupted fluency failures from a child and did so frequently (1985b). The frequency of occurrence of fluency failures in the children affected the frequency of interruptions by the mothers. When a child was fluent, mothers interrupted minimally (2% to 3%). When a child was disfluent, mothers interrupted frequently (15% to 18%).

All children produced fluency failures when they interrupted a mother. Approximately 1% of a child's interruptions occur when they are speaking fluently. Over 5% of a child's interruptions coincide with some form of fluency failure. It is not surprising that a child interrupts with some type of fluency failure because interruptions are commonly associated with the initiation of an utterance and stuttering usually occurs at the beginning of an utterance. The fact that stutterers experience more fluency failures would make their interruptions more prevalent. Teaching preschool stutterers more appropriate ways to take turns may reduce the cycle of interruptions associated with fluency failures.

In terms of the rate at which mothers spoke (Meyers & Freeman 1985c), mothers of stutterers were significantly faster in their talking to all children (5.48 syllables per second) than mothers of nonstutterers (4.96 syllables per second). Interestingly, the mothers of nonstutterers tended to speak faster to stutterers   (5.11 syllables per second) than to nonstutterers. This is further evidence that a child's stuttering influences the mothers' rate of speech in a reciprocal or bidirectional manner.

Newman and Smit (1989) varied the speech style of an adult during conversations with four different, normally-developing preschool children to determine if the speech production of a child (rate, interruptions, and fluency) was influenced by an adult (who varied the length of response time). If the adult used a longer response time (3 seconds), the child would increase in response time. When the adult used a shorter response time (1 second duration), the child would respond more quickly. Speech rate did not change in either the adult or the child as a function of increased or decreased response time latency. Two subjects, however, were influenced by the adult's response time latencies in terms of the amount and types of fluency failure produced. If the response time latency decreased, the subjects experienced more fluency failure. If latency increased, the subjects used fewer stuttering types of disfluency. The frequency of interruptions increased when the adult had a shorter response time latency because the child had limited time to respond to the adult. These findings also support the need for investigators to analyze reciprocal interactions to determine how the partner and child behaviour influence the rate of speech, the frequency of interruptions, and the amount of fluency failure produced.

Other studies have supported the unidirectional model and suggested that parents of stutterers differed in verbal interactions from parents of nonstutterers.   For example, Kasprisin-Burrelli *et al* (1972) reported that parents of school-age stutterers interacted more negatively with their children than parents of nonstutterers. Specifically, parents of stutterers were critical, dictatorial, threatening and interruptive. Mordecai (1979) found that parents of preschool stutterers exhibited more negative verbal profiles than parents of nonstutterers. Parents of stutterers interrupted frequently, not allowing their children to answer questions. Parents of preschool nonstutterers expanded on the child's utterances more frequently and were generally more positive in their verbal interactions. By having mothers (of stutterers and nonstutterers) interact with their own and unfamiliar children in a bidirectional and interactional manner, Meyers and Freeman (1985a) observed that mothers of stutterers and nonstutterers engaged in similar types of positive and negative verbal interactions no matter who the child partner was. Researching both directions of the interaction (between a child stutterer and partner), alters the way in which we believe parents are the sole contributor to the child's stuttering behaviour.

Fluency Failure When Talking to Parents

The next question regarding interactional research had to do with how much fluency failure was produced by preschool children (stutterers and nonstutterers) when they spoke to mothers. Was it possible that levels of fluency failure were influenced by the mothers' verbal interactions (i.e. interruptive patterns, fast speaking rate, negativity, and/or excessive questions)? There were no significant differences between the children interacting with different mothers with regard to fluency measures (Meyers 1986). There were, however, differences between stutterers and nonstutterers in the types and the amount of fluency failure produced. Quantitatively, stutterers emitted more fluency failures than did nonstutterers talking with different mothers. Qualitatively, stutterers had more stuttering types (part-word repetitions, prolongations, and tense pauses) and the nonstutterers used more normal types of disfluency (word repetitions and revisions). These findings are important in that a) stutterers were identified differently from nonstutterers in terms of the amount and types of fluency failure produced, and b) the mothers' verbal interactions did not contribute to the child's level of fluency failure.

There was the possibility that stuttering levels vary when children converse with other listeners (besides mothers). Mothers have been studied more frequently because in the area of child development, we know more about mother-child interaction than other relationships. Recently there has been more concentrated developmental research in father-child (Cath *et al* 1989; Clarke-Stewart 1977; Lamb 1977) and peer-child (Vandell & Wilson 1987) relationships. Meyers (1990) contrasted the verbal interactions between preschool stutterers and father, mother, and peer partners. In the experimental setting it was observed that mothers, fathers, and peers were similar in some ways and different in others in verbal interactions with stutterers. Parents questioned stutterers more frequently than did peers. Parents were also more positive towards stutterers than were the peers. Peers were significantly more negative and made more general comments to the stutterers than did the parents. Fathers were more verbal in addressing the preschool stutterer than were mothers or peers. Clinicians have stated that parents of stutterers are quite negative. In this study, peers were more negative than parents.

No matter what type of verbal interaction (positive, negative, inquisitive, or imperative) a partner produced, stutterers produced very similar types and amounts of fluency failure (Meyers 1989). For the majority of stutterers the level of stuttering was constant (12% to 13%) talking to different partners. These findings were very similar to those reported earlier where the stutterers emitted 12.8% stuttering talking to their own mothers (Meyers 1986). In terms of the types of fluency failure, stutterers used more part-word repetitions (5% to 6%) and prolongations (5% to 6%) than other types of fluency failure.

Fluency failures in preschool stutterers were not associated with specific parental or peer verbal behaviors. In particular, significant differences between mothers, fathers and peers were not associated with any systematic increases or decreases in fluency failure. This is an interesting finding, especially in light of peers' significantly greater negativity. Apparently, the stutterers' fluency was not adversely affected by their peers' negativity or parents' frequent questions.

Observing stutterers from a bidirectional perspective (stutterer interacting with a partner and a partner interacting with a stutterer) has been quite informative. An interactional model has allowed us to observe parental behaviors that may contribute to a child's persistence of stuttering and analyze how the stutterer is affected by interactions such as rapid speaking rates, negativity, excessive questions, and interruptions. A bidirectional model has also been helpful in allowing researchers to observe what may increase and decrease the frequency of stuttering. It is possible that the preschool stutterer is not influenced by listener reactions like school-age stutterers who report fear talking to certain listeners (Bloodstein 1987). Also, it may be that certain situations influence levels of fluency failure. Talking with more than one listener, in situations where there is time pressure, and in unfamiliar situations may increase fluency failures in preschool stutterers. Future interactional studies should address the quantitative and qualitative aspects of fluency failure in various speaking situations where demands on the length and complexity of an utterance may influence the variability of stuttering.

A great deal of information has been gathered about the stutterer and parent interactional relationship. This knowledge has been incorporated into clinical practice in assessment, intervention and counselling in the approach to treatment. We will discuss that program next.

Implementing Interactional Research into Clinical Practice

Assessing Fluency Disorders in Pre-School Children

After forty years of Johnsonian practice of counselling parents of stutterers, clinicians have been uncomfortable referring, assessing, or treating the preschool stutterer. Interestingly, Johnson did not recommend to the medical and speech-language pathology profession to wait for a child to spontaneously recover. He advocated intervention for children identified as fluency-disordered.

There is another reason clinicians have been reticent to differentially diagnose young stutterers. This had to do with the issue of spontaneous recovery from stuttering. It has been estimated that 75% of the children between 2 and 5 years reportedly outgrow stuttering by age 16. Many clinicians take a conservative approach to intervention by withholding treatment for stuttering until the child is 6 years or older, or by treating the child for articulation or language disorders. Martin and Lindamood (1986) cautioned that in terms of clinical management, all children suspected of a fluency disorder after receiving a differential diagnosis should be treated because the true odds of spontaneous recovery at best are 30 to 50%. In the past 10 years, assessment tools for differentially diagnosing preschool stutterers have been developed, making it easier to determine which children spontaneously recover and which do not. Currently, clinical programs diagnose and treat preschool fluency disorders because of advancements in differential diagnosis.

The Gregory and Hill (1980) model has been adapted for differentially assessing stutterers from normally disfluent preschool children in many clinics. Every child suspected of stuttering is evaluated for a fluency disorder and is screened for concomitant articulation, language, voice, and hearing problems. In our program, the evaluation begins by observing the critical verbal interaction between a parent and child. Either the mother and the child, or the father and the child enter a toy-filled playroom. Ten minutes of free-play interaction between the

45

specified parent-partner and the child is videorecorded from behind a one-way mirror. The session is then repeated with the different parent interacting with the child. Direct parent-child observations are important for four reasons: to enable a clinician to make a subjective macroanalytic judgment concerning whether the child has a fluency disorder or not; to collect data that can be reliably used to microanalyze responses; to obtain a representative language sample from the child that can be used to analyze the quantitative and qualitative disfluency pattern; to reduce anxiety the child may feel before a formal fluency assessment begins.

Approximately 45 minutes is spent assessing language, articulation, voice, oral mechanism, and hearing. Fluency disorders are measured by making: quantitative measurements to determine how much fluency failures persist; qualitative measurements to note the types of fluency failure present; a severity rating of the fluency disorder.

The entire evaluation requires approximately two hours. Assessing a fluency disorder is determined using the mother-child/father-child interactional tapes along with at least two additional fluency measures (Adams 1980; Culp 1984; Riley 1981; Stocker 1977). If a child is considered normally disfluent, the child is re-assessed every 6 months for several years. If a child is classified language impaired, the child is enroled in language therapy and fluency is stabilized through language intervention. If a child is considered fluency disordered, the child is enroled in direct treatment and the parents receive counselling. There have been 45 preschool evaluations for stuttering since 1985. Twenty percent of the children were considered *normally disfluent*. All the others were considered stutterers (6.67% *mild*, 48.89% *moderate*, and 24.40% *severe*). Thirty boys (7 *normally disfluent*, 2 *mild*, 16 *moderate*, and 5 *severe*) and 15 girls (2 *normally disfluent*, 1 *mild*, 6 *moderate*, and 6 *severe*) were evaluated.

Upon graduating from the Fluency Development Program, a child is assessed every 6 months for at least 5 years. These six month visits are critical. As evidenced by Table 1, nine children were diagnosed as being normally disfluent and have not become stutterers. For the 25 children who received treatment and graduated, 23 children have remained fluent. The remaining children are being treated for a fluency disorder.

Table 1. Follow-up evaluations on 32 children considered fluent speakers including normally disfluent children who were not treated and stutterers who received treatment and graduated as fluent speakers from the program.

FOLLOW-UP EVALUATIONS						
Initial Diagnosis	< 6 mos	6 mos	1 yrs	2 yrs	3 yrs	4 yrs
NORMALLY 3 DISFLUENT	2	1	3	-	-	
STUTTERERS:						
MILD -	1	1	-	-	1	
MODERATE 3	3	7	-	-	-	
SEVERE 2	3	2	-	-	-	

Routine check-ups allow a clinician to determine if a child continues to develop fluency skills or has relapsed and warrants additional intervention. The parents feel a sense of relief that the clinician is taking responsibility for monitoring the child's fluency development.

The evaluation process allows a clinician to observe the stutterer and family from a bidirectional perspective. After evaluation the stutterer receives intervention for the fluency disorder and the parents engage in counselling to alter behaviors that may contribute to the continuation of a child's fluency disorder.

Intervention with Pre-operational Pre-school Stutterers

While our fluency development program has combined components of successful and established treatment programs for preschool fluency-disordered children, two innovative additions are: a) Piagetian cognitive experiences are coupled with direct practice of slow, smooth, and effortless speech production; b) ongoing guidance is given to improve the quality of the parent-child verbal interactions (described later in the counselling section of this chapter).

Piaget (1926) posited that in order to understand the cognitive abilities of a preoperational child, an investigator must discern the cognitive structures underlying the individual's actions through repeated observation. Piaget assumed that cognition was a process that included maturation, sequential stages of development, environmental experiences, social influences, and the child's own active participation in development of thought. He described the preoperational child as *centered* indicating that the child's reasoning processes were perceptually bound. That is, the preoperational child fails to detect more abstract or invariant relations among objects because he is distracted by the perceptual or spatial properties of objects (Gelman & Baillargeion 1983).

Although Piaget reported that preoperational children failed standard conservation, classification, and seriation tasks, several researchers have taught preoperational children to successfully conserve, classify, and seriate information (Gelman 1969; Rosch *et al* 1976; Shatz & Gelman 1973). Children in our program are taught to speak continuously, effortlessly, and smoothly (known as *Easy Speech*) through the child's ability to conserve and classify information.

The preoperational child is not as conceptually developed as an older, concrete operational child or an adult who stutters. It has been an effective strategy to present to a preschool stutterer animals and demonstrate their actions in order to teach fluency enhancing techniques such as *Easy Speech*. Touching, feeling, and thinking about concepts of fluency are stressed through animal illustrations that children can readily comprehend. Four adjectives *slow, fast, smooth,* and *bumpy* are discussed during easy speech. *Slow* is defined as stretched speech production which maintains the suprasegmental features of intonation and stress. The *slow* concept is contrasted by discussing racehorse or *fast* speech. Racehorse speech is considered swift, rapid, and becomes unintelligible when we talk too quickly.

Smooth is defined as the continuous ease of speech production which has a gentle, even, and rhythmic flow. *Smooth* is contrasted with *bumpy* speech, which is irregular, displaced, choppy verbalization which resembles syllable repetitions or prolonged, stuttered speech.

The racehorse can also be used to illustrate fast and bumpy speech. For example, the racehorse moves so quickly and *buh-buh-buh bumpy* that his legs get all tangled up. The racehorse must slow down to unravel his tangles before he moves along. The point that is stressed is that the racehorse cannot continue to race quickly because he has to rest frequently which causes him to be inefficient and lose energy. The turtle moves along slowly, smoothly, and efficiently. The clinician models the effortless speech of the turtle and the bumpy speech of the racehorse. The story teaches the child a more effective and efficient way to speak (or to win a race with easy speech).

Communicative turn-taking activities are also an important component of therapy. Earlier research (Meyers & Freeman 1985a) suggested that fluency-disordered children interrupt frequently and do so experiencing fluency failures. For the preoperational child, taking turns is a very abstract concept. In order to understand turn-taking principles, the child is introduced to *Mr. Turn-taker*. Mr. Turn-Taker is an appealing stuffed animal that is held while someone is talking. Children learn that when they have possession of Mr. Turn-Taker it is their turn to speak and they will not be interrupted. When the clinician is talking, she also has access to Mr. Turn-Taker. When a child forgets and interrupts, verbal reminders to take turns are provided by the clinician. Sometimes children use 30 seconds of silence before completing their turn. Children need this time to execute lengthy and complex speech patterns and motorically produce fluent speech production. Learning to take turns allows the child the opportunity to take as much time as needed to respond fluently.

After slow, smooth, and turn-taking rules are explained, each child listens to a story read by the clinician in a very slow manner. The story is then repeated slowly, but this time the child is encouraged to provide one or two word responses. For instance, if the clinician is reading a story about the *Three Bears*, the clinician will point to a bear while the child stretches out the word *b-e-a-r*. If the child responds slowly or smoothly, the clinician reinforces the fluent response, models the word again, and explains what was good about the child's response (i.e. whether it was slow or smooth). The story is then continued in this structured manner. Within one story the child will have approximately 25 attempts to speak with controlled fluency.

Activities are used to encourage the child to use one- or two-word utterances in a slow and deliberate manner. The word level is selected on the basis of where the child can successfully produce fluency. Thus, an individual therapy session may begin with a structured activity requiring only single word responses if that is the level at which the child is fluent.

The session usually ends with a different story which is read slowly by the clinician with a follow-up explanation of the speech rules. All sessions are tape recorded for later analysis. The clinician records baseline data for fluency, number of utterances spoken and average length of utterances produced for every session. Then, progress can be charted and shared with the parents. It is the responsibility of the clinician to select a level where the child can begin to integrate the motor planning necessary to speak fluently.

Producing longer utterances and speaking under pressure are included in the long range goals of the therapy program. *Mr. Pressure*, a fast-talking, bumpy, inconsiderate turn-taker is introduced to the child when fluency has been established in the clinic. *Mr. Pressure* is another character introduced to assist children in understanding environmental pressures that can influence their levels of fluency failure. Children recognize that sometimes in the environment people will talk fast. Fluent (i.e. Easy Speech) talkers must practice activities that will assist them in not being influenced by extraneous pressure (e.g. fast talking, interruptions, negative verbal reactions, and/or questions from others). The clinician holds up a mask - Mr. Pressure - and talks fast, interrupts, and criticizes. The child usually thinks this is funny and tells the clinician to stop talking like the racehorse. After the child learns to maintain fluency and recognize Mr. Pressure, the mask is removed and the clinician will spontaneously insert pressure throughout the session. The child continues to tell the clinician to speak slowly and smoothly when pressure is perceived.

Intervention requires the clinician to assume certain responsibilities for ensuring that the child speak fluently. First, it is important for the clinician to model Easy Speech throughout the entire session. Second, the clinician must refrain from asking questions that will elicit lengthy and complex responses from the child. If a question is necessary, it should require a simple, short, and rote response thus preventing spontaneous conversational interaction and potential disfluency. Third, the clinician must plan activities that will elicit short responses that discourage the child from talking spontaneously. Fourth, the clinician must provide appropriate reinforcement for fluency throughout the session. If the child stutters, the clinician will withhold reinforcement and repeat the child's utterance using a) an explanation of what should be done to facilitate talking smoothly/slowly, b) a slow speaking model, or c) a model of the exact word, phrase, or utterance for the child to practice correctly. It is also important for the clinician to monitor reaction to the child's stuttering. Subtle moments of directed attention to the child, averted eye gaze, increased rate of speech and/or other nonverbal behaviors should be minimized.

The first hour of easy speech is spent in individual therapy with the child's own clinician. The second hour is spent in group therapy with 4 to 8 fluency-disordered children and an easy speech teacher assisted by student-clinicians. Individual therapy begins at a level where a child can successfully maintain fluency. If a child comprehends the slow concept more frequently than the smooth concept, then the rule *slow* is practised more rigorously during individual therapy. Group therapy provides a structured, fluent, and supportive atmosphere where children watch and model each other speaking fluently. Table 2 outlines activities and the time line for individual and group fluency intervention.

Table 2 Individual and group therapy sessions for children. Activities and time line for completion of the program.

Individual Activities

Storytelling (10 mins.). 2 or 3 Fluency Therapy Activities (25 mins.). Quiet Fluency therapy activity (15 mins.). Total time 55 min.

1 to 2 word structured utterances (4 weeks). 3 to 9 word structured utterances (4 weeks). 5 to 6 word structured utterances (4 weeks). Spontaneous, unstructured utterances (4 weeks). Structured utterances while introducing pressure and continued conversation (2 weeks). Unstructured pressure and continuation of spontaneous conversation (4 weeks). Unstructured pressure, continuation of conversation, parents each to prepares a separate, 5 min. activity (4 weeks). Prepare child for graduation: child skips a week of therapy and, if 93% fluent the following week, 2 weeks are skipped, then 3, then 4. If fluency is maintained, child graduates (12 weeks). Total time-line 38 weeks.

Call 3 months later to discuss child's progress (12 weeks).
Three months after phone call, child comes to clinic for re-evaluation (12 weeks).

Group Session Activities

Quiet interactive fluency activity (10 mins.). Active interactive fluency a (15 mins). Snack time (20 mins.). Quiet interactive fluency activity (5 mins.). Total time 50 min.

(Group format and activities are usually the same. *More fluent* children do more talking in unstructured situations while the beginning children stay at a very structured level.)

The intervention programme has summarized the child's active participation as a learner of fluency. The parent's role in the child's acquisition of fluency is also important and will now be discussed.

Counselling with Parents of Preschool Stutterers

Counselling attitudes have in the past been influenced by the Johnsonian hypothesis that stuttering develops as a result of the abnormal parental reactions to the fluency failure. Evidence to support this theory was based on interviews with parents and the finding that parents were responsible for the original diagnosis of the disorder. Johnson speculated that parents were overanxious, perfectionist, and unrealistic in terms of their standards for speech production. Working from these assumptions he counselled parents to refrain from criticizing, correcting, or reacting negatively to the child's speech. Other researchers went as far as to conclude from questionnaires, interviews, and rating scales that the parents of stutterers were neurotic and outwardly ambivalent, rejecting, overprotective, and dominating towards their stuttering children (e.g. Feldman 1976; Grossman 1952; Kinstler 1961). Although the basic premise of the Johnsonian theory has been strongly challenged and disproven, clinicians, pediatricians and teachers continue to counsel parents to alter negative interactions without conclusive direct evidence that parents contribute to a child's stuttering.

Counselling is offered to parents in an attempt to improve the stutterer's communicative environment, and as a consequence, reduce the chances of stuttering. Counselling recommendations have not been based on empirical investigations but on two assumptions. The first is that family members, acting as listeners, respond in ways that increase the likelihood of stuttering. The second is that family members and significant others within the environment share the same type of inappropriate listener response patterns. It may be, however, that not all listeners respond in a similar manner. For example, not all parents of stutterers exhibit negative behavior when interacting with their preschool stuttering child. It is the responsibility of the speech-language pathologist to objectively determine what negative behavior each specific parent displays during the evaluation process. Then counselling strategies may be implemented to meet the individual needs of each parent attending counselling. Comprehensive counselling and direct intervention experiences should be provided for the parents of fluency-disordered children. Parent behavior is assessed during the initial fluency evaluation when the parent and child are interacting in the free-play setting. Negative parental behaviors are quantified and ways to speak more positively to stutterers are discussed during counselling.

According to Luterman (1984) contemporary counselling is defined three ways. First, counselling is an educative experience occurring between two people. Second, it is problem-centered and allows for expressing feelings. Third, it encourages growth from both the counsellor and the client. In order to provide an educative, problem-solving, affective experience for parents, behavioristic and humanistic counselling principles are followed. Behaviorist counselling addresses observable parental behaviors that need modification, defines easy-speech terminology, and provides a communication forum in which parents exchange ideas and give specific examples which facilitate fluency in their children.

We define behavioristic counselling as the process in which a counsellor identifies certain parental behaviors that need to be modified during the initial parent-child interaction observation. Behavioristic counselling provides a structured framework for parents to become active at recognizing and changing behavior. For example, Meyers and Freeman (1985c) reported that mothers spoke very rapidly to young stutterers. A child's stuttering may create an uncomfortable feeling for a listener that potentially results in rapid speech production from the listener. Starkweather *et al* (1989) have parents slow down their rate of speech in order to provide a better speaking model for their fluency-disordered children. A behavioristic counsellor would not tell parents to *slow down*. Instead, the counsellor would design activities that would provide practise time for parents to learn how to slow down. Parents who have a naturally slow rate would provide models for parents who need practise. Behavioristic counselling is designed to provide instruction and practise to modify behavior. The counselling is instructional, straight-forward and unemotional.

The behavioristic counselling program covers many topics and these are re-visited more than once. Continued discussion on some topics lasts several weeks. Individual topics are presented according to the pace the parents select. For example, if a parent continues to discuss and ask questions regarding discipline, then discipline would continue to be a topic of discussion. Topic of focus continues until the parent group acknowledges that they are open to discuss a new topic area. These are outlined in the 10 sessions below.

Session 1. What is fluency?
The initial session describes what fluency is so parents can focus on positive attributes of speaking. Slow rate, continuity of speech, and ease of conversation is discussed. Fluency is contrasted with audio samples of normal disfluency and stuttering. (This topic area usually lasts 2 to 3 weeks.)

Session 2. What causes fluency disorders?

Parents discuss theories thought to cause stuttering. Parents share what they believe caused their child's stuttering. The goal is for parents to feel some sense of relief that they are not cause or at fault for their child's stuttering. (This topic area usually lasts 1 week.)

Session 3. Observing fluency at home.

Parents are given a homework assignment where they observe three situations in which their child is using fluent speech. Parents write down where the child was, what he was doing, who he was talking to, what he was trying to say, and how long he was fluent. The clinician and parent discuss carry over of fluency into other situations. The counsellor shares with each parent what specific therapeutic activities have facilitated fluency in their child. (This topic area usually lasts 2 to 3 weeks).

Session 4. Observing disfluency at home.

Parents are given a homework assignment to observe three situations in which their child is highly disfluent. Parents discuss their homework assignment concerning where they noticed disfluency, what the child was trying to say, to whom was the child speaking, what did the child actually do when speaking became difficult, how did the child react to the disfluency, how did the listeners react to the disfluency, how did the child react to the listener's reaction (adapted from Gregory & Hill 1984). Parents recognize that the child is usually disfluent in **pressured, unstructured situations**. They also understand that the speaking situation is too difficult for his current level fluency. (This topic area usually lasts 2 weeks.)

Session 5. Discussion of smooth versus bumpy.

Cognitive activities that can be implemented at home to reinforce the child's understanding of smooth, fluent speech are discussed. (This topic area usually lasts 1 week.)

Session 6. How to implement slow speech.

The purpose of teaching slow speech is so parents can provide an appropriate speech model for their child. By the time this session is implemented, the child is using slow speech in therapy. The parents soon recognize how difficult it is to speak slowly. They can appreciate the difficulty the children have had learning to talk slower. The child teaches parents which is a very positive experience. (This topic is discussed 1 week and followed up with practise activities for 3 weeks.)

Session 7. Discussion on child and behavioral development.

Many times parents want their child to talk at a level of linguistic complexity that makes it impossible for the child to maintain fluency. Therefore, parents learn about normal speech, language and behavioral development. Topics include a) what sounds are acquired at what age levels, b) what language skills (in terms of Form, Content, Use) develop at what age levels, and c) what age levels reflect certain attachment theories. Parents need to know what expectations are appropriate for their developing preschool child. (This topic area usually lasts 4 to 5 weeks.)

Session 8. Discipline.

Discussion typically emphasizes being consistent when discipline is needed, setting limits on child's actions but not feelings, and being a good listener when child is expressing feelings. Parents share actual situations occurring at home that they would like modified. Three rules are employed which are a) we do not harm property, b) we do not harm ourselves, and c) we do not harm others. (This topic area usually lasts 4 to 5 weeks.)

Session 9. Developing turn-taking skills in children.

One problem commonly associated with fluency disorders is that the parent and the child do not take designated turns talking. Frequent interruptions are made and subsequent disfluency is apparent when turns are not taken. The purpose of this activity is to assist parents in improving turn-taking skills. Parents are taught to count to two (Conture 1990b) before responding. (This topic area usually lasts 2 to 3 weeks.)

Session 10. Helping a child express feelings.

Parents are guided through active listening experiences that will promote discussion concerning communication of feelings between the parents and their children. (This topic area usually lasts 2 to 3 weeks.)

The humanistic counselling we provide establishes a relationship between parent and clinician so parents feel comfortable sharing feelings and attitudes concerning their child's fluency disorder. In humanistic counselling, the relationship between the counsellor and the client is equal - so both the counsellor and clinician assume responsibility for the course of therapy. Humanistic counselling is inspirational, imaginative, and intuitive.

The humanistic counsellor is specialized at recognizing the different processes parents experience after a child has been diagnosed as fluency-disordered. According to Moses (1985) denial, guilt, depression, rage, bargaining, and coping are healthy and necessary stages a parent and counsellor must work through towards understanding while the child is attending fluency therapy. Trained counsellors provide the empathy, non-judgmental, unconditionality and feeling focus that parents so desperately need.

Parents are given the opportunity to express and process the emotions they share as they face issues pertaining to stuttering. Disfluency places an emotional strain on all familial relationships. Through humanistic counselling, parents share coping styles and receive peer support - a support system that may have been otherwise unavailable to them if their child was diagnosed later on. Such groups can help parents acknowledge and work through the stresses of having a fluency-disordered child.

Results of The Treatment Programme

Since 1985, 45 preschool children have been evaluated. Over 71% of the children (51.1% stutterers and 20% normally disfluent children) are fluent. As for the rest of the children, 4.4% have relapsed after treatment, 20% are currently enroled in the program, and 4.4% have moved.

Table 4 Therapy outcome on 25 children.

Therapy	FLUENT GRADUATES			DISFLUENT GRADUATES		
	Mild	Mod	Sev	Mild	Mod	Sev
<6	2	3	2			
6	1	3	3		1	
9		4	1			
12		2	2			
24						
36						
48						
60						1

The average treatment period was 10 months. Children and families were seen once a week for two hours. The time spent in treatment, the number of successful stutterers, and the number of unsuccessful stutterers are presented in Table 4.

Ninety-two percent of the children enroled in the intervention program have graduated and have remained fluent. Eight percent (2 females) of the children enroled in the intervention program have graduated and have relapsed. Most of the successful children have been younger (2 - 5 years) and have been stuttering less than a year (8 - 12 months).

The program outlined in this chapter has been quite successful. Many research findings are now known about stutterer-partner interactions and how these interactions potentially affect treatment outcomes. There is more to learn about how interactions may influence the fluency development of children who are at risk to stutter. The last section of this chapter describes a longitudinal research programme implemented to observe fluency development and failure in children who are at risk to potentially stutter.

A Prevention Programme

Early intervention with preschool stutterers is considered a *secondary prevention* effort. Primary prevention infers that the clinician is stopping something from happening before it starts. The way most speech-language pathologists have defined prevention is as identifying and treating the problem after the disorder has developed. The Asha Prevention Committee (Kilburg *et al* 1988) and centres for the study of epidemiology term this *secondary prevention* or *early intervention*.

In order to prevent stuttering, a clinic would have to follow at-risk parent-infant and parent-toddler verbal interactions longitudinally. A primary prevention effort would be to observe fluency development in toddlers who may have a genetic and/or environmental predisposition to stutter. By collecting quantitative and qualitative data on at-risk children, eventually clinicians will be able to counsel the parents and teach some compensatory skills that will lead their children through normal fluency developmental phases.

One obvious group to consider at risk would be those children who have familial incidence of stuttering (Williams 1987). We have collected data on 9 at-risk toddlers who have relatives who stutter. The children are observed every 6 months beginning at 6 months of age. In this study, two children have begun to stutter and a third child is highly disfluent. A female child began stuttering at 20 months of age. Initially she was videotaped at 13 months of age and exhibited two part-word repetitions while playing with her father. At 20 months of age she was emitting lengthy part-word repetitions and prolongations on every other word. This child qualified as an at-risk candidate because her father, paternal grandmother, paternal great aunt, male cousin, and 3 year old sister were all severe stutterers. During a one hour play period with the mother, a clinician spoke very slowly and provided a good model for the child to follow. The mother was encouraged to verbally interact in the same manner. The child is now 4 years of age and has remained fluent since the mother began implementing an easy speech program at home.

The second child was 30 months of age when he began to stutter. He too had family members who stuttered. He spent six months in intensive therapy and is currently considered a fluent speaker. His progress will be monitored every six months until he is school age. The third child is being monitored at 6 month intervals and the parents have been encouraged to speak slowly at home. She remains highly disfluent but uses mainly whole-word repetitions and revisions. Currently, the parents are less concerned about her fluency failures.

Summary

Observing stutterers from a bidirectional, interactional model has allowed us to observe verbal behavior that may contribute to a child's persistence of stuttering and analyze how the stutterer is affected by interactions such as rapid speaking rates, negativity, excessive questions and interruptions. A bidirectional model has also been helpful in allowing observation of the development of stuttering.

Our research has shown that investigations into the parent-child communicative interactions critical to the development of stuttering has assisted in the understanding of diagnosing, treating, counselling, and preventing fluency disorders in young children. Individualized and group instruction for young stutterers, group counselling for the parents of stutterers and a diagnostic follow-up program for at-risk children has been provided based on clinical research.

Acknowledgements: Special thanks to Lee Woodford who has spent a great deal of time and effort contributing to the Fluency Development Clinic and the student-clinicians who provide services to the children and their families. This work was partially supported by Psi Iota Xi, the ASHA Foundation, and the US Department of Education (G008400756).

Chapter 4

Parents and Their Pre-School Stuttering Child

Willie Botterill, Elaine Kelman and Lena Rustin

Introduction

Is there anything new to write about the management of childhood stuttering? Have not all the theories and issues been recorded and discussed? The literature is replete with programmes and models to equip even the most inexperienced clinicians with the means to tackle this enigmatic population. Yet there remains uncertainty, reluctance, and caution within the profession borne of fear that intervention may be actually harmful to the child, causing any disfluency to become worse rather than better. Many writers testify to the dramatic improvement in the preschool child's fluency when early intervention takes place. Prins (1983) exhorts us to expect a rapid generalised improvement in fluency when things that provoke communicative uncertainty in the child's home environment are being altered. Bloodstein (1987) in his review of the literature writes that *reports of success in therapy with young stutterers are common, and there appears to be a widely held belief among clinical workers that the disorder is usually easily treated in early childhood* (1987: p. 399).

So, why when the evidence for intervention is so positive do large numbers of preschool stutterers remain in the *review* files, waiting until they are experiencing difficulties at school, with heightened awareness and numerous other complicating factors? Riley and Riley (1983) state that *delay in initiating treatment is serious because treatment is simpler, briefer and more effective with preschool children than with school aged children* (p. 43). We would postulate that clinicians would undertake the management of preschool stutterers if only they knew what to do. The literature is largely in agreement that parental counselling is an important component of intervention (Cooper & Cooper 1985; Riley & Riley 1983; Starkweather 1987) and many excellent pamphlets and books have also been produced to instruct parents in the management of their stuttering child (Conture & Fraser 1989; Byrne 1984; Irwin 1988).

The literature clearly describes the areas that should be considered when counselling parents and how parents can make changes. In his description of the *Demands and*

Capacities Model, Starkweather (1987) includes parents and siblings under the category of *Demands*:

> *Children have a natural tendency to use speech and language that is similar to that used by those they are talking to. Consequently, parents and siblings who talk rapidly inadvertently place a demand on a child to talk rapidly. Rapid turn taking and a fast rate both suggest to a child that there is little time in which to say what they want to say... Children's desire to match parental behaviour may also be seen in the level of language they use. When parents talk to their children using sophisticated language - syntactically complex and with an advanced vocabulary - the children try to use the same forms* (p. 78).

Clinicians may well know **what** to advise parents in the content of the counselling but there continues to be a shortfall regarding advice on **how** to effect change in parents' management of the child; that is, the method of counselling. Costello (1983) points out:

> *when one is trying to produce change in the family environment and the treatment/counselling is going on in the clinical environment, one is basically operating through advice and conversation...This kind of long distance, second order treatment, aimed at changing family members' behaviors beyond the confines of the clinicians's office, seems to be a rather distant and imprecise method of effecting change* (p. 73).

Our intervention is directed towards actively involving the parents with their child in the process of change. This chapter will provide clinicians with a framework for helping parents to become active participants in the process of recognising and changing behaviour.

Assessment

We no longer consider assessment to be a discreet phase in management that ceases once *therapy* begins. It is rather an on-going process that begins formally, and continues to be a part of therapy enabling the therapist to modify and refine therapy accordingly. Both parents of the disfluent child are required to attend for an in depth interview that may continue for 2 - 3 hours. The gathering of information helps us begin to understand the family systems, lifestyle, and prevailing communicative environment as well as the role played by the child and the disfluency within this setting. The disfluent child is interviewed separately at this stage.

The parental interview (Rustin 1987a) was designed for use with parents of disfluent children from age of onset to school leaving age, and has been described in some detail elsewhere (Rustin 1987a; Rustin & Cook 1983; Rustin *et al* 1987b; see also Chapter 1 where the parental interview is described and reproduced in the Appendix). However, for this age group there are areas of questioning which are perhaps particularly pertinent.

The first section of the interview is concerned with encouraging the parents to *tell their story*. Kelly (1955) reminds us that when we wish to understand the nature of the problem we should ask the participants to describe it. The questions encourage the parents to discuss their anxiety about the speech and other problems that may be causing concern. It often becomes clear that the speech is by no means the only or indeed the most pressing issue. Parents theories as to the cause of the stuttering help us to discern their understanding of the disorder and perhaps their view of the likely outcome of therapy.

The general medical background along with the family history and the child's developmental history will help us discover any genetic or physiological predisposing factors and give some impression of the physical capacities of the child in question.

An in depth exploration of the family and environment helps us to establish an understanding of the physical and emotional demands that may be contributing to the child's difficulties.

Finally, the interrelationships between family members are explored in an attempt to establish the nature and pattern of the relationships that exist within the family. As discussed earlier, demands from within the family or from within the child may significantly affect the development of fluency.

The formal assessment of the disfluent child is usually conducted concurrently with the parental interview. If it is necessary to do this on a different occasion the child is interviewed prior to the parental interview. The assessment includes measures of stuttered words per minute, words spoken per minute, percentage stuttered words and types of disfluencies. These are taken from tape or video recorded samples of speech over a range of activities. The child's speech and language skills are also assessed to determine whether there are complicating underlying motoric and or linguistic difficulties.

The stuttering child is then interviewed to help the therapist explore his/her view of their difficulties, which may or may not agree with that view expressed by their parents. We continue to be surprised at how many young disfluent children are able to verbalise their concern regarding their speech. For example, a young four year old girl was quite clear that it was *very hard* for her sometimes when *the words won't come out* whilst others remain relatively unperturbed. Some time is then spent with the child trying out various strategies which may directly or indirectly increase fluency. These may include the therapist reducing their rate of utterance, reducing the linguistic demands or indeed practising an easier way of speaking (Rustin 1987a).

Finally, a differential diagnosis between normal non-fluency and the disfluencies that are characteristic of early stuttering will be made based on information from the parental interview and the type and number of stuttering behaviours recorded.

Making this diagnosis can be problematic and controversial (Hayhow 1983). However researchers have identified several criteria which are generally accepted as indicative of early stuttering:

1. A high frequency of repetitions (two or more) on instances of part word syllable repetition (Gregory & Hill 1984).
2. The presence of the schwa vowel in place of the target vowel in syllable repetitions (Van Riper 1982, Gregory & Hill 1984).
3. Production of three or more within-word speech disfluencies (e.g. sound/syllable repetitions and prolongations) per 100 words of conversational speech (Conture & Caruso 1987).
4. Struggle behaviour - the likelihood of chronic stuttering increases with the amount of effort that a child puts into speech production (Starkweather 1987).
5. Explicit concern expressed either by the parents or by the child (Conture & Caruso 1987).

The physical and emotional environment of the child are also important considerations. Prins (1983) mentions erratic household routines, unsettling time pressures and insufficient time spent alone with the child, as being sources of environmental stress. Riley and Riley (1983) discuss the relevance of parents high expectations of their children, and indeed children's high expectations of themselves as further contributors to environmental pressures. The clinician will now be in a position to make decisions regarding intervention.

All the information gathered is brought together at the conclusion of the interview and the therapist should help the parents make sense of the whole problem, discussing with them all the factors that have emerged during the interview that may put this particular child at risk. The clinician should draw attention to any genetic or physiological predeterminants that exist as there is considerable evidence that stuttering runs in families and stuttering children frequently have co-occurring speech and language difficulties (Andrews *et al* 1983).

Intervention Procedures

Those families where the fluency is determined to be within normal limits, and there are no other complicating or predisposing factors, may be advised to attend for counselling sessions to inform them about the nature and development of normal speech and to monitor periodically the development of the child's speech.

For families where there are signs of early stuttering and/or there are other predisposing factors, a more directive approach would be required. It is at this stage that we are further interested in the nature of the interaction between the parents and their child. Starkweather (1987) shares Conture's view that stuttering results from a complex interplay between the child's environment and the skills and abilities the child brings to that environment.

In order to look at this aspect more fully a task called **talking time** is set at the end of the interview for the parents to complete at home before their next appointment. The task is negotiated with each parent who makes an individual commitment to spend three, four or five minutes; four, five or six times per week playing with their child. They are instructed that **talking time** is their task and they will have to ask their child to help them with it, and should negotiate with the child a time that is mutually convenient. At the appointed time the parent should ask the child to choose a toy or something they would like to play with, for example, cars, Lego, dolls house, but it should not be reading or TV. The parent and child then go into a room, close the door so that they will not be interrupted by others, and once settled, time the task and encourage the child to talk by joining in with the activity. The parent should not make any demands or comment on the child's speech but should listen carefully to **what** is being said, not **how** it is said. When the time is completed the parent should thank the child for helping them with their homework and record in a notebook that the task has been completed making a few comments on how they felt about doing it (Rustin 1987a).

Parents should be reminded that the time limit is important and should not be exceeded, as it is the quality of time that is important rather than the quantity. The talking time is then set for two weeks to allow time for them all to become accustomed to the task. This exercise provides a routine framework for making changes in the future, ensures the commitment of both parents to therapy and also their willingness and ability to undertake tasks as instructed by the therapist. Any problems completing the task should be discussed fully with the parents and the child and the time rearranged if necessary. If the parents continue to be unsuccessful in completing the task, their ability to assist in the therapy process must be questioned, and they should be encouraged to return to therapy when they are more able to offer a firm commitment.

The following therapy procedures require the parents to be active and willing participants in exploring alternative ways of managing the disfluent child and assisting the development of fluency. Those parents who have completed the task return after two weeks for therapy. At the beginning of every session each parent is video recorded separately conducting a talking time session with their child for five minutes. This will provide the clinician with a basis for assessment of the parent/child interaction; from this treatment steps may be planned systematically. The discourse is analyzed in terms of the verbal content, its context, and a note is made of the non-verbal behaviour of the parents and the child. The focus is mainly on the parent's verbal and non-verbal behaviour, as research has shown that the model that the parent provides for the child will directly influence the levels of fluency. Newman and Smit (1989) suggest that some children as young as 4 years old are able to adjust one aspect of their speech when the speech of their conversational partner changes. Thus a child may attempt to emulate a parent who is using inappropriate verbal and non-verbal interactions. The clinician should detect all the fluency disrupting factors in the interaction, the most prevalent of which are described next.

1.   **Rapid Rate of Parental Speech**

A study by Stephenson-Opsal and Bernstein Ratner (1988) demonstrates that a reduction in maternal speech rate resulted in a substantial decrease in the disfluencies of stuttering children. Meyers and Freeman (1985) found that adults speak faster to children who stutter and Starkweather *et al* (1987) noted that an increase in rate was one kind of parental reaction to instances of stuttering. The clinician therefore will need to consider whether the parent's rate of speech is placing undue pressure on the child, which may result in an increase in disfluency.

2. **Poor Listening and Turntaking: Interruptions**

Meyers and Freeman (1985a) analyzed the interaction of disfluent children and highlighted the frequency of maternal interruptions. The clinician should note the number of interruptions that occur and the effect this has on the child's level of fluency. We have also observed that poor parental listening skills further disrupt the discourse with inappropriate interruptions that take no account of the child's contribution to the interaction.

3. **Parental Questions**

Adults frequently resort to repeated questioning in an attempt to stimulate conversation. However, Wood (1986) indicates that this is counter productive and that it is **commenting** that encourages verbal exchange. Continued questions put additional pressure on the child and increases the likelihood of a stuttered response. Parents also often fail to wait for the child's reply before presenting them with a further question.

4. **Adult Response Time Latency**

It is important that parents act as models for the child in respect of their response time latency (Newman & Smit 1989). If a parent pauses before responding to the child's utterance (increases the response latency time) the child will be more likely to allow themselves time before responding and therefore increase the likelihood of fluency (Meyers 1990).

5. **Syntactic and Semantic Complexity of Parent's Speech**

Haynes and Hood (1978) demonstrated that non stuttering children show more disfluency when producing modeled sentences of greater syntactic complexity. Thus if parents are presenting a verbal model to their **stuttering** child at a high level of syntactic and semantic complexity it is more likely that their disfluencies will increase. Parents also often attempt to discuss events that are unrelated to the activity currently occurring and therapy should be directed towards an appropriate level of language for the child that is related to the current activity.

6. **Directiveness**

Some parents become over directive in their play sessions organising the activities and dominating the verbal interactions. This is associated with poor observational skills and lack of attention to verbal and non-verbal cueing from the child. Andronico and Blake (1971) found that training parents in non directive play sessions with their stuttering children helped increase their fluency.

7.   **Non-Verbal Behaviour**

Close attention should be paid to parents non-verbal behaviour in the recorded interactions, as this may demonstrate negative attitudes. Lack of experience in playing one to one with their child, anxiety regarding their own abilities or behaviours, poor rapport, impatience, lack of warmth, difficulty relating to their child may be observed in their posture, positioning, facial expression, eye contact, intonation patterns, etc. The child would be *picking up* these signals which could cause adverse reactions.

The clinician should make a note of all the disruptors that occur during the video recording and then view the recordings with the parents, encouraging them to make any comments, particularly regarding their behaviour during the videoing and their feelings about it. At this point it is important to re-emphasize that the purpose of this exercise is to make some changes in the interpersonal communications that may assist the child in becoming more fluent. The clinician should then make some positive statements about the interaction and guide the parents towards **one** fluency disruptor that is either, something that they (the parents) have already drawn attention to or one that the clinician feels the parents would be able to tackle relatively easily. The rationale for making this kind of behavioural change and its implications are discussed with the parents. The clinician may wish to model the desired behavioural change for the parents, shaping and reinforcing their interaction as appropriate. The parents are then video recorded again individually trying out the new behaviour in a further play session with the child.

At the conclusion of the session the parents are instructed to continue practising the change and to monitor themselves and the child in the five minute talking time home practice, recording their activities on their homework sheets as before. On their return the following week this procedure is repeated; firstly to monitor, encourage and reinforce their efforts, secondly, to reinstruct or redirect where appropriate, and thirdly to bring into discussion another of the identified fluency disruptors with a view to making changes as before.

This process continues on a weekly basis for approximately one hour. The clinician should take care to praise and encourage parents' attempts to make changes and to help them see themselves as the agents of change. It is our experience that having worked through their initial discomfort (seeing themselves on video), they derive enormous benefits from being able to view their interactions with the stuttering child in a more objective manner. They often become very effective evaluators of their own behaviour. These sessions can incorporate discussions on a wide variety of topics that have either stemmed from this exercise or indeed from an issue that has emerged during the week. Topics can be diverse and may range from coping with eating problems or bedtime routines to managing *well meaning* but difficult Granny!

We would expect to continue these sessions once a week for 6 weeks. A longer period of approximately 3 - 4 weeks is then negotiated as a period of consolidation during which time the parents should continue to practice at home and return their homework sheets weekly for monitoring by the therapist. The therapist should reply to the parents on receiving the homework sheets, reinforcing and commenting as appropriate.

If there is an increase in fluency the family are encouraged to continue to monitor and practice with their child, returning homework sheets weekly for a further period of 6 weeks, with the proviso that if problems arise they should contact the therapist. The family then attend for review and if fluency is being maintained they are reviewed at three monthly intervals for up to two years.

In our experience the majority of families have not needed further intervention. However, in the event that the stuttering remains resistant to the modifications made to the child's speaking environment it would become necessary to employ direct speech modification techniques. The therapist should first establish an easier fluent speech pattern, by trying a variety of approaches; e.g. easy onsets stretched speech, slowed rate, running words together. We take a cognitive behavioural approach to the problem which requires that the child is involved in the process of discovery and that a common language is developed for describing the difficulties in talking and the strategies that alleviate them.

The chosen approach is then modeled and practised in structured activities that reduce the linguistic and semantic complexity, usually beginning with one word utterances or short phrases of two or three words. This base line fluency should be firmly established before increasing, in easy stages, the linguistic complexity of the tasks. Time is also spent identifying and discussing the **stressors** that make talking difficult, like people interrupting or wanting to go too fast. Games and exercises are structured towards teaching the child to resist these stressors as fluency increases. The parents are also involved in the process of learning fluency control techniques so they can provide an appropriate model for the child when difficulties occur at home. A much more detailed description of this approach may be found in Rustin's (1987a) *Assessment and Therapy Programme for Disfluent Children.*

Speech and Language Problems

Disfluent children often present with underlying speech and language impairment (Bloodstein 1987). This may pose interesting questions for the researcher as to possible common causes, but gives a clear indication to the clinician of the importance of treating both presenting problems. A motoric or linguistic breakdown might well contribute to the maintenance of disfluency. Wall and Meyers (1984) suggest that some children may have particular problems with one or more levels such as in lexical selection, in sentence structuring, in co-ordination of respiration and vocal tract movements, or in co-ordination of spatial and temporal integration of articulatory gestures.

A therapy programme that combines fluency training and language remediation should be carefully structured so that the fluency practice is focused at a lower level of output than the language therapy; for instance, if a child is at a three word level in expressive skills, fluency training should be conducted at a two word level. Similarly, clinicians should be aware of the dangers of focusing on output in a language disordered child. As Starkweather (1987) warns children receiving language therapy should be closely monitored, and if stuttering begins to occur, therapy should be altered to reduce pressure on the child's performance.

Illustrative Case Study 1

John, aged four years, was referred by a speech therapist for specialist consultation, as his mother was extremely anxious about his continued disfluency. Both parents were interviewed and the case history revealed a family history of stuttering on the fathers side and John's father presented with a moderate stutter which he felt did not present any hindrance to his daily life. The parents reported some difficulty in their marital relationship but did not relate this to John's difficulties.

John presented with a moderate stutter, featuring part word repetitions, prolongations and struggle behaviour. He was able to verbalise the difficulties he experienced in communicating and expressed a desire to overcome the problem. His speech also featured a phonological delay with impaired intelligibility. His cognitive and language skills were superior to his chronological age.

The management of this family consisted of a three pronged approach:

1. Initially four counselling sessions were arranged with the parents to discuss their marital problems and examine the implications of these for John and his difficulties.

2. Video recording sessions focusing on the interaction between each parent and John.

3. Individual treatment of John's phonological delay.

The video sessions with both parents were conducted over a period of 6 weeks. Aspects of behaviour that were highlighted were:

Father: excessive questioning, rapid rate of speech, tense body

posture, short response latency time.

Mother: physically passive role in play sessions, inappropriate positioning,

failure to follow child's verbal cues.

At the end of the 6 week period John's disfluencies had decreased markedly and the contrast in the video recordings was very reinforcing for the parents. John was then seen for a further 6 sessions for the management of his phonological delay. He made good progress and the parents were advised to maintain the changes they had achieved and were reviewed at three monthly intervals. The clinician felt that John was particularly at risk of further disfluency due to the strong family history. Two years later, John's mother contacted the clinic to report a dramatic increase in the frequency and severity of disfluency. It transpired that John had just changed schools to attend a private school with an emphasis on academic achievement.

John was taken back into therapy for a 6 week period when he was taught how to modify his speech to achieve fluency. John grasped the concepts easily and implemented the changes in his speaking pattern, supported by his mother who also learned and practised the technique. The disfluency decreased and John was instructed in the need to modify his speech when difficulties arose. Almost a year later John is continuing to maintain his fluency.

Illustrative Case Study 2

Mary was referred at 3;06 by her GP following persistent pressure from her mother who was highly concerned about the disfluency. The case history revealed a stable but lively family setting, no family history of stuttering but some delay in Mary's early language development. Mary presented with a moderate stutter featuring part and whole word repetitions and prolongations. She was able to describe her difficulties with *getting words out* but was not particularly anxious about it. Mary had a younger sister of 20 months who was lively and vocal; demanding much of the family's attention.

Some time was spent with the parents discussing the need to give Mary attention and the opportunity to talk without being interrupted by her vociferous sibling. Apart from establishing a talking time, turn taking was discussed in order to reduce the pressure on Mary when she was communicating with her parents. Six video recorded sessions were conducted when both parents concentrated on reducing their rate of speech, the levels of questioning and their overdirectiveness in play. In addition, Mary's mother focused on improving her listening skills during the talking time. At the end of 6 weeks Mary's fluency was within normal limits and 3 years later this level has been maintained.

Conclusion

The management approach which we have outlined enables the clinician to follow a structured programme of sessions aimed at helping parents change their behaviour and the communicative environment of the child to assist in the process of becoming more fluent. In some cases further therapy will not be necessary, for others it provides a sound basis for more direct work with the child's fluency, phonology or language as necessary.

Parent counselling may also be required in addition to these sessions to discuss issues that emerge in more detail or to deal with specific problem areas; such as marital discord, inconsistent management of the child, sibling rivalry, etc.

The use of the video recorder is a vital component of this approach to intervention as it provides instant feedback for both parents and therapist. It is a powerful and effective tool in therapy which can be illuminating, revealing and reinforcing to both the parents and their stuttering child.

Chapter 5

Using Families To Help The School-Age Stutterer: A Case Study

A.R. Mallard

Six years ago I was introduced to family intervention in stuttering therapy (Andrews & Andrews 1983; Rustin & Cook 1983). Not only was my horizon broadened by experiencing new ideas, but my philosophy of what was important in stuttering therapy for children changed. I hope the following information will serve as a similar stimulus for you. This chapter will illustrate the efficiency that can be expected when working with cooperative parents and describe how a group-designed parent program (Rustin 1987a; Mallard 1989) can be used with elementary-age school children on an individual basis.

In 1981 at Southwest Texas State University we sought to upgrade our training offerings in stuttering therapy for children. The motivation to make changes came after a three year project conducted in the public schools of San Antonio, Texas (Mallard & Westbrook 1988) that demonstrated conducting stuttering therapy twice a week following the itinerant model (ASHA 1984) without parental involvement was not optimal in effecting long range changes in school children. After investigating stuttering therapy programs in Washington, California, Virginia, New York, and London, England, the decision was made to introduce the English program (Rustin 1987a) at our clinic. This therapy approach appeared to be the most comprehensive in meeting the needs of the stuttering child, while at the same time exposing graduate students to the complexities involved in stuttering therapy in a time-efficient manner.

The uniqueness of this therapy lies in its use of social skills training, which has been used for some time in the field of mental health (Trower *et al* 1978), but is a relatively new concept in the management of communication disorders (Rustin & Kuhr 1989). The therapy model is based on the assumption that intervention with individuals who influence the communication environment of the stuttering child is the critical component in the treatment of stuttering children. Our treatment plan is based on the following assumptions:

    a) communication is a social skill; any therapy for stuttering children must take into consideration the social environment in which the child communicates;

b) parents determine the communication environment of their children at home and the teacher determines the communication environment at school;

c) the communication environment of each child is unique;

d) the family's structure, as well as the structure of a classroom, and methods of interacting are unique and must be understood if carry-over is to take place in the normal speaking environment, be it at home or at school;

e) therapy must address two issues - first the modification of the child's speech production to produce improved speech, and second the use of appropriate social skills so newly acquired speech patterns can be used in the normal environment;

f) therapy must address the desire and/or ability of the parents and teachers to carry through with activities that will allow the child to use newly acquired speech skills;

g) the parents must experience as much of the therapy as possible so that realistic expectations concerning the eventual progress of the child can be developed;

h) family dynamics that might initially appear to be extraneous to the management of stuttering emerge and should be addressed during therapy.

Most of our stuttering children are seen on a two week, intensive program each summer. We require that the stuttering child, both mother and father, and all siblings over the age of six years participate. A total of 46 individual topics are covered.

I want to add an important note before you read further. The preceding paragraph described how we usually conduct stuttering therapy in our clinic. Please do not think that you have to conduct an intensive program like we do, or like Rustin (1987a) does, to use this therapy concept. The nice feature of working with families is that concepts can be applied to groups on an intensive basis or to individuals on a non-intensive basis. The clinician has the flexibility to adjust the topics and schedule to fit individual needs.

I also want to encourage you to think about therapy somewhat differently than you probably have in the past. It is important not to be locked in to one service delivery model. The results from our school service delivery study (Mallard & Westbrook 1988) indicated that changes are probably going to have to be made in the way stuttering children are managed in the school setting if accountability (Mowrer 1972) is to result. My experience suggests that the problem of stuttering is much too complex to conduct therapy on an individual basis (clinician and child only). We must involve the people responsible for the child's communication environment from the beginning of therapy if the child is going to use what is learned in a meaningful way. Involvement does not mean talking with the parents infrequently about what is happening in therapy. Involvement means working with the parents, child, and teacher **as a unit** so reasonable decisions can be made to help the child when problems occur.

To use the therapy described in this chapter effectively, you must branch away from what Andrews & Andrews (1989) refer to as the **individual** model of service delivery. The individual model is characterized by four features:

1) the interactive system is the client (child in this case) and the clinician;

2) change is looked for only in the child;

3) the primary intervention is with the child;

4) change occurs during the session.

The therapy approach described here is **systemic** (Andrews & Andrews 1989), which contrasts with the individual model in that:

1) the interactive system is the child **and** a circumscribed group of people who interact with the child, have influence on the child, and are concerned about the problem;

2) change is expected in the individual **and** in the interactive system;

3) change occurs in the natural environment;

4) the primary intervention **is with the interactive system**.

You are probably conducting most of your therapy following the individual model. I want to encourage you to try the systemic approach.

Using the Family: An Illustrative Case

The remainder of this chapter outlines the step-by-step procedure that was used with the family of a stuttering boy (6;0). The parents and stuttering child were seen first and the teacher was involved afterward. Schedule conflicts precluded working with the teacher at the same time. I would encourage you, however, to involve the teacher as much as possible for the entire therapy process. This family was chosen for this chapter because the insights gained by the parents, child, and classroom teacher illustrate perfectly how efficiently therapy can be conducted when the parents and school personnel work together under the guidance of the speech-language pathologist. Names and other identifying information have been changed to preserve anonymity.

Therapy included six weeks of homework assignments prior to the initiation of 15 individual, 30-45 minute, therapy sessions with the child and family. Two meetings with the classroom teacher, one at the beginning of the academic year and one at the end, illustrate how the teacher worked with the child **during regular class time** to accomplish transfer of new speech skills.

The first step is to conduct an interview and assess the child's speech and language skills. A two hour, comprehensive interview with the parents outlines the development of the child, the child's current level of functioning, the interaction patterns within the home, and a description of the history and current status of the stuttering problem. A thorough case history forms the basis of therapy for this program. It is from the history that the clinician begins to understand the dynamics of the family, how the problem of stuttering relates to communication patterns within the home, and the stuttering child's place in the family structure (Rustin & Cook 1983). (See Chapters 1 and 4 for detailed discussion of the initial interview and parental interview.) A complete speech, language, and hearing assessment of the child is also conducted at this time.

John, age six and in the first grade, was referred to our clinic by the parents. He had received speech therapy for one year in the school setting (once a week for 20 minutes) and the parents were not pleased with his progress. He attended speech therapy the last half of kindergarten and the first half of the first grade. The parents decided to seek outside assistance when it was reported by John's teacher that he cried when he had to go to speech therapy.

The assessment was conducted in the spring, followed by the initial homework assignments. Therapy started the following September, when John entered the second grade, and was concluded by mid-term of the spring semester. The teacher became involved when John entered third grade.

Case history information revealed that the stuttering began at about age three. The problem would *come and go* and the severity ranged from *mild to severe*. The parents reported that the problem was worse when John was attempting to *explain something*. They also indicated that the stuttering tended to be worse at the beginning of the school year, during moments of excitement or fatigue, or during periods of *allergy attacks*.

The stuttering pattern was characterized by prolongations and repetitions of initial sounds of words. Secondary features included enlargement of the eyes, talking on residual air, loss of eye contact, and elevation of fundamental frequency. The frequency of stuttering ranged from a low of 10% during echoic speech to a high of 48% during monologue. The stuttering frequency was observed to be higher during the *formal* assessment phase of the evaluation than during spontaneous play at the conclusion of testing.

The family history was largely unremarkable. John had a brother (1;6). The parents indicated that John's stuttering seemed to be more of a problem to them than to John. They were concerned, however, about the advice they had been given by the previous speech-language pathologist. The parents had been told not to discuss stuttering with John: they were basically to ignore the problem. According to his mother, *John knows he stutters. He asks me sometimes why he doesn't talk right. What am I to say, "I don't know?" I've been told not to talk about it.* In addition, they were not to discipline him by physical means, such as spanking. They were also told that they should make every attempt to listen when he talked regardless of what they were doing. This was a problem for the parents because John tended to monopolize conversations with lengthy stories and long stuttering blocks, ranging from one second to as long as 20 seconds. His mother stated:

> *How can I pay attention to him when he is talking and I am driving the car? He continues to talk and talk, stuttering more and more with each sentence, and I am not suppose to say anything until he finishes. I can't listen to him and drive the car at the same time. Anyway, by the time he finishes his story, I forgot what he was trying to say and, for his sake and mine, I can't ask him to start over...It seems as if he knows he has me when he is talking and he is not about to give me up.*

John's mother indicated that they were led to believe that the parents were probably responsible for John's stuttering. Consequently, she had developed *considerable guilt.* The parents were not involved in the treatment process and had little contact with the clinician following two case conferences at the beginning of the school year.

At the conclusion of the interview we bring the parents and child together to give the parents an assignment called *Talk Time* as described in detail in Chapter 4.

The importance of this assignment cannot be overemphasized. The routine of conducting talk times that the parents and child establish at this point form the foundation on which all future home management will be conducted. It addition, the talk times give the clinician an indication of the parent's desire and/or capability of following instructions.

A total of six weeks of talk times (thirty sessions) were completed prior to the initiation of therapy. These assignments were conducted during the latter part of the spring semester and early summer. The child was not, and preferably should not be, enroled for therapy during this time. The clinician received the homework assignment sheets and responded accordingly. The following description outlines the observations made by the parents during the talk times.

During the first week, the parents noted that John tended to stutter more when he became excited. They stated that his speech *seemed better this week than the last week*. The stuttering was reported as *gone* for most of the second week but seemed to return as John became tired.

John had an ear infection during the third week and the parents said his speech was worse. He was tired so mother *did not push him*. The talk times were conducted only during the mornings this week because his speech *tended to be better in morning*. The report from the fourth week was significant. The parents commented on the detail John used in his talking - the fact that his *stories go on and on*. Speech was described as *fairly good this week*.

John was reportedly upset during the fifth week due to an accident on a seesaw and an incident that happened on a field trip to a museum. He apparently got off the seesaw early and caused it to crash, hurting another child. John's mother reported that his speech *became worse* following this incident. During a class trip to the museum, John asked the guide a question. Apparently there was considerable stuttering. The guide did not let John finish and this upset John and his mother. The mother made a significant statement describing this incident. She said she wanted to interrupt and talk for John but *just kept my mouth shut to see what would happen. It killed me but I hung with it*. The mother reported John's speech as *terrible* on the way home.

The sixth week was apparently bad so far as stuttering was concerned. Both mother and father noted facial grimaces in John's stuttering. The stuttering tended to be worse when trying to relate a series of events. It was stated that John's speech seemed to be erratic - that it *goes from very good to horrible in the same paragraph*.

The decision was made to begin therapy when school started in the fall. It was further decided that the speech pathologist in the school who the parents had seen before would not be involved in the process.

The remainder of this chapter will discuss each therapy session. The intent is to provide you with a sample of the topics that were discussed. You are referred to Rustin (1987a) for a complete description of the rationale for the therapy sequence and topics covered.

The Therapy Program

Weekly therapy began in September. All therapy sessions were conducted with both parents and John. It was agreed that if all three family members could not meet, then therapy would be cancelled. A different topic was covered each week with homework. Each therapy session would begin with a discussion of the homework for the previous week. The physical set-up of the room was always the same: the chairs were arranged in a circle. Note that because of the talk times, the parents had progressed from saying nothing about speech to developing a routine of observing, documenting speech activities, and establishing a time to think about speech during the week in the home environment.

Session 1 (September 16): The first session was an orientation and discussion of expectations. John said he would like to stop stuttering - *It takes me hours to say some words*. A discussion was conducted concerning when John stutters the most. John said he stutters when he gets excited; mother said it was when he is trying to relate a story. A discussion occurred about what happens during stuttering. John said *something happened* in his throat. Another conversation began about what John wanted his parents to do to help him with his speech. The father said he wanted the clinician to tell him what to do. The mother also did not know what to do. She said she would do *about anything*.

The session ended with a discussion of expectations. The mother expected the therapy to be honest - to tell her what could be done and how the environment could be changed if necessary. John expected us to help him stop stuttering. The father expected the therapy to help them help themselves. The homework was to begin the talk times again since they had taken a break from this task during the latter part of the summer.

Session 2 (September 23): All agreed it was good to start the talk times again. This session was about observation. A list was developed on the board that identified what could be learned by observing other people. They identified such factors as mood of the individual, whether the person was comfortable or not, whether a person is hot or cold, the kind of day the person had, season of the year due to the clothes the person is wearing, etc. The homework assignment was to make one observation of another person two times during the next week. Talk times were to remain the same. In addition, the parents were each asked to complete the *Disfluent Behavior Checklist* (Nelson 1982) in which they were to identify characteristics of John's stuttering.

At the end of the session it was noted that John tended to look at the father more during conversations. He also tended to stutter more when talking to the mother.

Session 3 (September 30): After a discussion of the homework assignment, the topic turned to observations made during the week concerning John's stuttering. Each discussed what had been observed in the speech pattern.

After this discussion, John and a student went to another room to observe his speech in a mirror. The mother, dad, and clinician practised stuttering like John. The mother made willing attempts at duplicating the stuttering pattern. The father, however, refused to try. He said he became *nervous, felt hot, and froze*. He said his mind went blank. The father was asked how he believed John felt when he (John) was called on to talk, knowing he would stutter. The father indicated he had not thought of that before but he believed John would not want to talk. The father was eventually able to imitate the stuttering pattern.

It was explained that the idea of therapy was to allow the parents to experience stuttering as the child did. The parents would then be able to respond to John's questions from experience. The father was immediately able to see why avoidance is such a problem for stutterers when he, the father, tried his best to avoid stuttering in the clinical environment. It was explained that therapy did not always include tasks that we like. If John was to progress in learning controlled speech in the normal talking world, he would have to eventually learn to control his speech in talking situations that were difficult, and that he probably did not like.

John and the student returned to the room. John's mother and father practised stuttering and John watched and made comments as to whether or not their stuttering was like his. John indicated that his Dad's stuttering was more like his, which was most reinforcing for the father!

The homework assignment was for the parents to stutter like John during the talk times this week. In addition, the parents were to have one instance of disfluency with a stranger during the week.

Session 4 (October 6): The discussion of the last week's homework was revealing. John commented that his father did the best last week with the stuttering during talk time. He commented, *Dad can copy my stuttering the best. Mom just sort of didn't stutter hard enough.*

The parents, as do most people who complete this assignment for the first time, both reported being uncomfortable with voluntary stuttering. Both were embarrassed. The father reported that his face turned red. The point was made by the clinician that the feelings they experienced were probably the same as John feels when he is called on to talk. The mother asked John how he felt when he stuttered. He responded, *Bad.* She said she never realized that, or even thought to talk to him about how he felt about his speech. Recall that she had been instructed previously not to discuss the problem with him.

The focus of this therapy session was listening. A brainstorm session (listing all possible ideas) was conducted concerning the following question, *How do you know when a person is listening to you?* Fifteen items were written on the board.

The homework assignment was to continue the talk times and play a listening game three times during the week. In addition, there was to be a family discussion as to who talks, listens, and interrupts most in the family.

At the conclusion of this session, the parents were told that speech work would begin next session. The mother indicated that John continues to talk when she asks him to be quiet. She said it seemed to be a discipline problem but was afraid to make him be quiet when he talked too much due to the instructions they had received from the previous clinician. She was reminded of her statement about being controlled by John when he was talking. She said it would be nice if she could make him mind when he is *driving me crazy with his speech and stuttering.* It was agreed that John's continuous talking was indeed a social skills problem and should be treated as she would treat similar kinds of problems. She asked if it was okay to make him *hush* when she did not want to listen to him or when it was not convenient for her to listen (such as driving the car). When she was assured that her suggestion was quite acceptable, she stated, *We are going through a tremendous deprogramming process from the other clinician. We are so relieved that our lives do not have to revolve around the way John talks and that we can discuss it openly.*

Session 5 (October 14): The session began with John stating that the stuttering had been less this week, and this was verified by his mother. It was agreed that mother does most of the talking at home.

This session began speech training. The family was told that the most important thing was to keep therapy as simple as possible. We wanted to identify two or three techniques that the family believed were important and concentrate on those. A brainstorm session took place on the following question, *What happens to speech when we talk slowly.* Eleven items were listed. **Slow speech** was practised for the duration of the therapy session, with each family member taking turns and being criticised by the clinician. The homework assignment was to do talk times in slow speech this week. Slow speech was to be used only during talk time, not during other times during the week.

The practising clinician should begin to see the importance of using the established talk time routine as the key to accomplishing carryover activities at home. It is the talk time activity that provides the structure for home practice and parental involvement.

Session 6 (October 28): The homework discussion focused on slow speech. The parents indicated that the teacher had noticed John talking at a slower rate at school. Recall that work had not been conducted on carry-over activities and John had already begun to transfer. The mother indicated that it was difficult for John to use the slow speech during talk times this week since, in her opinion, he had to think of what he was going to say as well as monitor his speech. She and her husband decided that it would be best to select topics that were somewhat easy for John to discuss.

The mother also went on a field trip with John's class. Some of the children asked her why John talked the way he did in John's presence. She told them about stuttering and then, on the way home, discussed it with John as to the appropriateness of the response. She felt good about the manner in which it was handled and the discussion that occurred on the way home. She and her husband also noted some self-correction attempts by John during the week. An important point was made concerning the possible expectation of using slow speech all the time. It was explained that it was not natural for John to talk slowly: it was natural for him to stutter. Therefore, it would be an unreasonable expectation for him to monitor speech all the time.

As can be seen from the above paragraph, this was an important week for therapy progress. Keep in mind that this was just the sixth therapy session and only one session had concentrated on speech change. John had transferred on his own. The parents had used their observation skills to gain insight about the stuttering and then made the proper decision about how to proceed. The mother made the proper response to questions about John's speech and the problem had become desensitized to the extent that a discussion about the *therapy session* during the field trip took place. This is the kind of progress that is seen in most families when the parents and child are trained to deal with stuttering at the same time.

The therapy session this week involved praise. The distinction was made between verbal and nonverbal praise. A brainstorm session took place focusing on different ways to respond to praise. The homework was to continue talk time with slow speech. The parents were to praise one of John's behaviours and note how the praise was accepted.

Session 7 (November 4): The homework indicated that John was able to use the slow speech during talk times this week with no stuttering present.

The session this week involved **problem solving**. This session differed in that John was to use slow speech during the problem solving and throughout the session if possible. The goal of this therapy is to get the family to see stuttering as a problem that can have many possible solutions. We want the child to understand that the key to solving the stuttering problem is to identify what option(s) he or she wants to put into effect and then help the parents let the child experience the resulting consequences.

The first step was to solve a non-speech problem. The problem solved during therapy was one suggested by the father. He said, *My problem is that there is not enough light at the end of the day to finish my work*. The homework was to conduct a problem solve at home that was not related to speech.

Session 8 (November 11): The importance of problem solving and letting the child take responsibility for his problem was the discussion that initiated this therapy session. John indicated that he believed his speech was worse this week. He indicated that he wanted to talk fast but knew he would have problems if he did. The comments from the parents on the homework sheets were that John was not as careful about slow speech this week but still he was more in control than before.

The problem solve this week was, *What do we do when John is stuttering?* Thirteen suggestions were mentioned. It was decided by John that he wanted his parents to tell him to *talk slow* when he was having difficulty. It was decided that the mother was responsible for Sunday through to Wednesday and the father for Thursday through to Saturday. There would be no reminders on Sunday. Each parent was allowed six reminders per day.

Note that is was not sufficient for John to tell his parents what he wanted them to do. A specific plan had to be developed on how and/or how many times he wanted them to remind him. It is important that the child be in charge of this discussion when making these decisions. If the child is ever to take responsibility for managing **his problem**, then he must be leader in making decisions about his speech. The plan must be agreed to by all concerned, however. It would not be fair for unreasonable demands to be made by the child and expect the parents to comply.

An equally important point needs to be made about the parents at this point in therapy. When the child makes decisions about what is to happen in speech therapy, the parents must be willing to follow the child's lead. One of our most important findings to date is that children make faster progress when parents follow their (the children's) lead in deciding what is to be done about stuttering, not when the clinician or parents are telling them what is best. This may sound difficult to accept at first. Our experience suggests, however, that when the children learn the variables involved in speech change, they are perfectly capable of deciding how they want to use them and the role of each family member. We have had some children who want their parents to do nothing about the stuttering. Other children, like John, are very specific about what role they want their parents to play.

One of our most striking examples of this point came during the first year of our therapy program. An eight year old boy was asked, *What do you want your father to do to help you with your stuttering?* The boy, looking at his father, replied without hesitation, *I want you to change your job.* The father was perfect in his response, *Tell me what my job has to do with your stuttering.* The boy said, *You travel a lot and are gone from home most of the time. I think it would help my speech if we could spend more time together like we have this week and talk more. My speech seems to be better when we are talking together during talk times.* The boy and the father were able to work out a plan whereby the father would call home more frequently than in the past and have talk times on the telephone when it was not possible for them to be together. This information, let alone this solution, would not have been known if the clinician or the parents were the ones telling the child what was best for him.

Session 9 (December 9): This session concerned John's lack of turn-taking skills. The mother seemed to be frustrated and indicated (again) that this was a major problem at home. The father agreed and said that some days he had a headache by the time John goes to bed from all of John's talking. It was agreed by all parties that it was okay for the mother or father to tell him to stop talking when it was necessary. It was also emphasized that the

83

parents had to be in control of the home and that John must learn appropriate social skills, whether he stuttered or not. The mother indicated again that they were trying to overcome two years of *walking on eggshells*. It was difficult for them to be assertive when it came to making John change his speech or other discipline matters at home.

Session 10 (January 22): John was ill and the parents requested a meeting even though we agreed at the beginning that the entire family had to be present for each session. The parents reported that John was in a very disfluent period. Mother said that she was stopping him now when he is talking too much and that he was responding in a positive manner. John's positive response made her feel better about herself. We reviewed the social skills we had discussed to date. The parents were encouraged to problem solve as much as possible. We talked about directive/facilitative conversational styles. Both agreed they tended to begin too many conversations with questions. The homework was to change one directive statement to a facilitative statement and observe the reactions.

Session 11 (January 27): John and the clinician worked on speech rate. John was disfluent on almost every word at the beginning of therapy. A stack of word cards were used and the parents and John practised saying words slowly and feeling the smooth movement. Speech rates were defined as one as slow rate, two was normal rate, and three as fast rate. After practising with individual words, he told a story and changed the rates as he talked. He was able to monitor this very well. He said he did not like to talk at rate three - *I stutter too much*.

During therapy he tried to tell long stories and was very disfluent. It was decided that the parents would conduct a family meeting (a time when the entire family sits down to discuss an issue or solve a problem) this week in which the long stories and continual interruption would be problem solved.

Session 12 (February 10): The family decided that John did indeed make his stories too long and furthermore, it was not polite to expect others to wait. It was also discussed that his stuttering added to the problem. The family agreed that it would be fair for the parents to tell John to be quiet when he was talking too much and that John could finish the sentence he was saying. They reported that this plan worked well for the first week and agreed to continue with this plan for the next few weeks. John said he liked the praise his parents gave him when he quit talking when asked.

Therapy this session emphasized articulating plosives with reduced contact. Again, a stack of word cards was used. Individual words were practised, contrasting hard articulatory contacts with easy contacts. The words were used in a sentence toward the end of the session. Slow speech was used frequently and John was able to achieve good practice with plosives.

Session 13 (March 31): The mother reported that speech was *severe* this week. John continued to talk excessively in the car. She also indicated that his speech was probably at its worse when in the car. A decision was made that John would limit his talking in the car until he could either talk in *short stories* or use slow speech and stutter less.

This session emphasized starting the voice gently on voiced sounds. The Visipitch was used. Mother, Father and John all tried to obtain easy onsets. John was the most accurate. The last part of the session emphasized practising slow speech with all targets (specific speech skills) being monitored and changed. Homework was to continue talk times and manipulate targets as the talk time progressed.

Session 14 (April 3): The father said that he had offered John 25 cents if he would use his slow speech while riding in the truck. He said John turned him down because not stuttering was not worth the effort for just 25 cents!

All agreed that we had accomplished about as much as possible and that practice was needed at this point. The parents indicated they were comfortable with their role and that open communication was taking place in the home regarding the stuttering. Observations from past therapy confirmed this statement. This session was devoted to determining where we go from here. Three decisions were made: (1) future efforts should involve the larger family, including grandparents; (2) John would attempt to catch himself one time per day and either talk slowly or change a hard word to an easy word; and (3) the teacher needed to be involved in the therapy process.

Involving the Child's Teacher

I want to turn now to the involvement of the classroom teacher. Frankly, when we started working with teachers, I was surprised at how quickly the teachers adapted to the problem solving concept of management. The children in the classroom have also been a part of the process which makes it easy for transfer to take place.

Recall, the teacher for this year had not been part of therapy. The parents told the teacher about John's stuttering at the beginning of the year and requested a meeting. The decision was made to meet two weeks after school started. The meeting would involve at least the teacher, John, the mother, the speech-language pathologist at the school, and myself. The principal of the school also asked to be part of the meeting. The parents requested that he not be enroled in speech at school since they had completed therapy at the university. The primary focus at school would be with the teacher, not necessarily the speech-language pathologist at the school. This was different a service delivery model and the principal was not sure about the concept.

The meeting was opened by John telling the group about his stuttering. He described what he did during speech that resulted in stuttering. He also identified (and demonstrated) what he must do to help himself speak more fluently.

I then explained that we had two problems that we wanted to address. One was John's uncontrolled stuttering. It was explained that he knew what to do to help his speech but that he did not always want to use the skills. It was further explained that John realized that it was not fair for the class to have to wait for him when he was stuttering out of control. The next problem was that John tended to talk too much when telling a story. He needed to say what he was going to say in a few words and stop.

The classroom teacher (Mrs. Smith) was then invited to help John with his speech and it was explained to John that there were two problems she could help with. First, John was asked what he would you like Mrs. Smith to do to help when he was stuttering out of control but she did not have the time to listen. John said he wanted her to raise her finger by her side (he demonstrated). *When she does this, I will either stop talking or use my slow speech.*

Mrs. Smith demonstrated that she understood what John wanted her to do when he was stuttering out of control and she wanted him to stop. Mrs. Smith then demonstrated what John had asked. He wanted her to place her hand by her side, not in front. He demonstrated and they practised until she understood exactly how he wanted her to signal.

The next problem the clinician introduced was when was John telling stories that are too long. Mrs. Smith was asked if she would like to help John with this, and she agreed. John was asked what he wanted Mrs. Smith to do when he was telling a long story and it was time for him to stop. John said that he wanted her to raise the same finger but this time place her hand in front of her, not by the side. John demonstrated for the teacher and Mrs. Smith showed that she understood what to do.

Following this discussion, Mrs. Smith and John practised. John demonstrated voluntary stuttering with long stories and Mrs. Smith practised raising her finger. John practised completing the sentence and stopping or using slow speech to control the stuttering. The meeting lasted about thirty minutes.

Mrs. Smith was encouraged to contact the parents if she had questions. The meeting ended with everyone feeling a sense of direction and good about their roles.

A significant event occurred after the meeting. The principal took me aside and said that he had never seen such a demonstration and wanted to know how it could be incorporate into handling more problems in the school.

I was in contact with the parents during the year. We had one refresher meeting during the fall. At the end of the school year, we had another conference with the same personnel involved. This time the teacher was in charge. She indicated that she had to signal John three times during the year. According to Mrs. Smith, John just seemed to know when he was talking too much or needed to use slow speech and took appropriate action. She said *John and I knew when he was working on his speech. We added a new twist. When I saw him making an effort to help himself, I would wink at him. He would wink back.* She indicated that there had been no problems during the year and felt comfortable talking with John about how he wanted to handle such activities as oral reports. Her closing comments were, *John has worked hard on his speech this year and I have seen progress. Be sure to involve his fourth grade teacher in the same way. This was a piece of cake!*

John is presently not enroled in speech and is in the fifth grade. He is reportedly doing well in school and speech has not been a negative factor in his personal or school lives, according to his parents and teachers. The most significant improvement, according to the mother, is that he has learned to take turns during conversations.

I hope this chapter serves as a motivation for you to work with families of stuttering children. You have seen that 14 sessions with the parents were all that was needed to teach the family how to manage. The actual number of sessions will of course vary from between families but our experience suggests that 14 is about right when working with individual families. When the family is trained to make daily decisions about management, and the classroom teacher is working with the child in a manner that is suitable to the child and teacher, then stuttering children can be removed from the daily roles of the speech-language pathologist for the majority of the school year.

Chapter 6

Intensive Management of the Adolescent Stutterer

Lena Rustin, Willie Botterill & Frances Cook

Introduction

The treatment of fluency disorders in adolescence continues to concern speech clinicians. Virtually all adolescent stutterers have a relatively long history of disfluency and as the final years of their schooling approach both they and their parents become increasingly concerned about their future. Stuttering is a disorder of childhood with onset as early as 18 months, new cases continuing to arise up to 9 years of age. The available evidence on the development of disfluency points to the increasing risk of the problem becoming chronic as it persists into the adolescent years. Andrews *et al* (1983) reviewed the research concerning *spontaneous recovery* and concluded: 75% of those stuttering at age 4 will have recovered by 16 yrs; 50% of those stuttering at age 6 will have recovered by 16 yrs; 25% of those stuttering at age 10 will have recovered by 16 yrs. Although this indicates some tendency for stuttering to disappear of its own accord, this becomes increasingly less likely in adolescence.

The adolescent is at risk of developing the chronic problem associated with adult stuttering, where it may be seen as a major obstacle to the formation of close relationships, as well as seriously affecting work and career prospects. The problem of adolescent stuttering is further compounded by the very process of adolescence. Radical and disturbing changes are taking place in the transition from childhood to adulthood: development of self awareness and self doubt; the first experiments with independence and decision making; concerns about sexuality in terms of both bodily changes and mental set; increasing demands of school; changes in relationships with parents, family - and perhaps most importantly, peer relationships. During this time most adolescents are learning to accept their strengths and their weaknesses, experimenting with decision-making, taking risks and coping with the inevitable failures that occur in pursuing their struggle for independence. Stuttering adolescents may quickly learn to blame their failures on their stuttering, thus avoiding the painful but important experience of having to take personal responsibility for their own actions.

We have noted that many adult stuttering clients, by attributing their problems in adolescence to stuttering, have not developed the skills required for normal social interactions. There are well documented difficulties in the transfer and maintenance of fluency which may be linked with these deficits in adolescent experiences. Indeed speech clinicians are showing an increasing interest in the possible psychological factors which may be contributing to the problem of maintenance of fluency. Perhaps the stutterer as an adolescent was quick to blame failures on the speech problem rather than learning to accept true strengths and weaknesses.

There are strong indications that parents play a crucial role in treatment of childhood stuttering (Conture 1982, 1990b; Gregory 1984; Rustin 1987b; Starkweather 1989) and that this role changes as their child reaches the nexus between childhood and adulthood. During childhood the parents usually exercise their authority in family matters. This may cause trouble between the parents and the adolescent, notwithstanding the fact that it may be prompted by the parents' continuing concern for the child - particularly where a problem such as stuttering persists. However the adolescent is still part of a family unit and the clinician must be prepared to learn about and understand the family systems in order to involve the parents in a practical, logical and agreed way.

Our aim is to encourage a partnership that will assist in the development of independence, growth of decision making and ability to negotiate areas of disagreement. Stuttering therapy for the adolescent therefore needs to consider the difficulties the client is experiencing with their personal transition to adulthood and this must take place within the context of the family unit. Other authority figures (teachers, relatives, etc.) also loom large in the life of the adolescent client. In many cases adolescents are endeavoring to establish their own autonomy in a reasonable way, but in some cases there is a rejection of or rebelliousness towards every person seen as an authority figure - including the clinician.

The intimate relationships with peers is often problematic for adolescents and it is the early relationships between parents and children that are often considered responsible for these difficulties. Button (1980) suggests that by later adolescence this family influence is so firmly embedded that therapy should be specifically directed to *young adults*, rather than children locked into inappropriate relationships with their parents. Button also draws attention to the adolescents' desire to be *noticed* rather than *overlooked*, many preferring to get into trouble or become well disliked than not to be noticed at all, and therapists should be aware of the role stuttering may play in this context.

Thus there are a number of problems in the treatment of adolescents which require consensual solutions. Many speech clinicians are faced with the dilemma of treating adolescents either through an extension of treatment programmes designed for children or alternatively, by scaling down treatment approaches employed with adults. Perhaps the most fundamental point emerging from any reputable therapy programme is the necessity to tailor treatment to the individual's needs. To create uniform treatment packages which are applied in a standard way to a group of individual stuttering clients is to miss the essential nature of speech disfluency - its individuality. Some disfluency is found in otherwise quite healthy and psychologically stable adolescents; other cases of disfluency may be associated with rather severe social, emotional and learning difficulties. In all cases the breadth and specific content of therapy would need to be quite unique to the individual.

The aim of this chapter is to describe our comprehensive treatment programme which can be adapted for the needs of the individual following a wide ranging assessment procedure. The treatment programme maintains its flexibility throughout the clients progress. Changes occurring as a result of therapy, or new factors emerging during therapy, must be accounted for in order to achieve the best possible outcome.

Assessment

The assessment sets out to obtain a detailed case history of the family from both parents (Rustin 1987a) and the adolescent stutterer.

Parental Interview
Understanding the nature and patterns of relationships in the home makes it possible for the therapist and the client to use the family as an important resource in therapy. The parental interview lasts for between 2 - 3 hours (Rustin 1987a). This is the same interview procedure as used by Rustin in her programme and is used with families of stutterers from age of onset of the disorder to school leaving age (see the appendix following Chapter 1). During this time

we hear the parents view of their stuttering child within the family setting and have an opportunity to establish a relationship which we will draw on throughout therapy.

Adolescent Interview Assessment

It is vital to listen to and understand the problem from the adolescent's point of view. We ask many questions about school life, their performance and career plans as well as their feelings about teachers and peers. Home life is explored,including relationships with siblings and parents and their reactions to the stuttering. Their social life and interests within and outside the home are discussed. Particular time is spent asking questions about their speech - as we need to understand their theories about the cause of stuttering, their perception of the stuttering and how it occurs, what affects it and any control strategies they have developed.

An understanding of their attitude towards therapy is of particular value where there has been some experience of failure. We explore with them the implications of change: How would it be if they were fluent? What difference would fluency make to their lives? If there was just one thing they could change about themselves, what would it be - if anything? What strategies do they use to deal with problems?

Following the interview various assessments help us shed light on the specific nature of their speech difficulty. We video tape-record a standard fluency assessment (Rustin 1987) which derives a percentage of stuttered words (%SW), a stuttered word per minute count (SW/M) and words spoken per minute count (WS/M), as well as a qualitative description of the different types of stuttering behaviours. The British Picture Vocabulary Scale (Dunn & Dunn 1982) is routinely administered for screening other speech and language difficulties.

It is important that the therapist summarizes all the information gathered at the interview and makes decisions regarding the appropriate intervention strategy for that particular individual at that particular time. These are then discussed fully with parents and the adolescent. Care should be taken to explain that there is no cure for the problem nor one prescribed route to fluency, but a joint exploration of alternatives to enable the stutterer and the family to take charge of their problem. There are times when it may not be appropriate to offer a two week intensive course and other alternatives will need to be considered. Flexibility is demanded throughout therapy to take care of the needs of the individual, whether they are in group or individual therapy.

It is also necessary to ascertain whether parents are unwittingly colluding with the stutterer in using the speech problem as a scapegoat for the trials of adolescence, or may inadvertently sabotage therapy in order to maintain the *status quo* within the family.

In this chapter we are concerned with those stutterers who are able to participate and would benefit from an intensive course. The principle criteria for acceptance being an individual whose main problem is stuttering, who is actively interested in seeking help and is prepared to give up a significant part of the school holidays (often a major factor). Once accepted, they will be expected to attend for 2 weeks, on a daily basis (excluding weekends), for a minimum of 5 hours per day, plus group follow up sessions at 6 weeks, 3 months, 6 months and one year. Individual weekly therapy would be arranged as appropriate after the course. Parents would be expected to attend as required (minimum 2 - 3 days).

The Two Week Intensive Programme

There are three major components to the therapy programme:
1) Fluency control techniques;
2) Relaxation and social skills training;
3) Techniques from Personal Construct Therapy.

It is important to stress at this point that assessment *per se* will continue throughout the two week course and is seen as a fundamental to the therapeutic process.

Fluency Control

Participants on the course frequently state their desire to acquire fluency skills and share a belief with their parents that an improvement in their school work, behaviour, attitude, and social life would be the result. Experimenting with fluency control techniques helps the stutterer to adopt more realistic expectations of fluency. There is also a growing body of evidence that there are, at least for some stutterers, underlying physiological deficits affecting the co-ordination for the motor control of speech (Conture & Caruso 1987; Moore & Boberg 1987). Fluency techniques based on physiological modifications are therefore seen as an essential component of the course.

There are many programmes available that attest to the relative ease of establishing fluency (for example, Cooper 1984; Ryan 1974; Shine 1980); however the transfer and maintenance of this fluency outside the clinical setting is known to be a much harder task (Helps & Dalton 1979; Perkins 1973).

The first activity in teaching fluency is to encourage the group to find out for themselves, through *brainstorming*, a) the elements of normal speech production, b) the processes involved in the motor speech act and c) how this process breaks down during stuttering. The adolescents are then in a position to experiment with ways of controlling these elements and work individually, trying out their own personal fluency techniques based on their new understanding of the areas of breakdown.

This might include slowing down, softening sounds, easy onsets, thinking first, pausing, flowing words together, etc. The individual training programme works through graded steps in three modes - reading, monologue and conversation, to a criterion of two minutes fluency in each mode. Transfer activities begin at an early stage using simple verbal group games gradually becoming more complex and incorporating role play and outside assignments. Emphasis throughout is given to the concept that the ability to change the stuttering behaviour must be placed firmly in the hands of the adolescent with the therapist as facilitator.

Ideas and terminology from the group are used to generate group strategies and targets. Individuals are then encouraged to use those strategies and control techniques that assist them in being fluent. Adherence to a particular technique is not recommended but rather a problem solving approach may be used - *What actually is the problem here? What can I do to put it right?* thus leaving the stutterer to make decisions, and alter their speech in a way that is acceptable them. Fluency targets are achieved first in individual sessions and then increasingly in group activities, the overall aim being to help the adolescent gain a sense of control rather than achieving 100% fluency.

It is our view that part of the process of dealing with transfer and maintenance is in both the client and parents understanding that the fluency is not necessarily the answer to the problems of adolescence. This allows all concerned to look at the wider issues involved in an atmosphere of shared understanding which in turn helps the stutterer to take responsibility for his or her stuttering.

Social and Relaxation Skills

Rustin and Kuhr (1989) found that deficits exist in the social skills repertoire of adult stutterers that contribute to their difficulties in maintaining longterm fluency. Rustin (1984) demonstrated the long-term effectiveness of incorporating a social skills module into a two week intensive therapy programme.

The social skills of each individual are assessed using a standard check list (Rustin & Kuhr 1989) at the beginning of the two weeks to identify specific areas that will require training. These may range from very basic skills such as eye contact during a conversation, to much more complex interactional skills, such as making friends.

Particular attention is paid to seven specific areas of skills training: observation, listening, turn-taking, negotiation, relaxation, praise and reinforcing and problem solving. Considerable time is spent throughout the two weeks using skills training exercises (Rustin & Kuhr 1989), role play and role rehearsal, developing these to meet the needs of the individuals within the group. Each training session begins with a rationale and discussion related to the topic to be covered as it is essential that the adolescents see the skill as being useful in their own social world or it will immediately become redundant. The skills are taught using exercise video recordings, demonstrations and practice. This continues until the adolescents are confident and competent enough to complete homework tasks based on the newly acquired skill. These homework tasks are essential early transfer activities which will not only reveal difficulties that can be resolved with the help of the group but also, when successfully completed, will encourage all group members to greater efforts.

Observation

Many stuttering adolescents have difficulty maintaining eye contact and their poor observational skills often lead them to make incorrect judgments about the people with whom they communicate. Directing attention away from the stuttering towards other features of communication and observing the non-verbal behaviour of others alters the nature of the interaction, in a very positive way.

Listening

Adolescent stutterers are often so preoccupied with their anxiety about speaking that they fail to listen adequately. Instead they begin to anticipate the difficulty they may have in responding; as a result their responses are not only stuttered but also often inappropriate.

Focusing attention on what the other person is saying and teaching good listening skills such as acknowledging, reflecting back, self disclosures, etc. not only reduces some of the anxiety but also improves the quality of their interactions.

Turn Taking

Turn taking is an important feature in initiating, maintaining and ending conversation. Stutterers have considerable difficulty with this aspect of communication which is compounded by their poor observation and listening skills. Exercises to improve turn taking skills help the adolescent to become less preoccupied with their stuttering behaviour and to concentrate on the conversation in hand.

Negotiation

Being able to negotiate successfully is of particular importance to stutterers as it helps them to deal more successfully with peer relationships, parents and authority figures. Negotiation brings together all the elements of social skills training and prepares the adolescent for adulthood.

Good negotiators will be less confrontational and more able to assert themselves. This will enhance their ability to communicate with others and find mutually agreeable solutions to issues without resorting to stuttering, thus contributing to the long term maintenance of fluency.

Further problem solving and negotiation might be necessary in follow-up sessions to help various members of the family to negotiate with each other until a mutually acceptable solution to a problem is found. This would include encouraging and helping the parents to *let go* allowing the adolescent gradually increasing autonomy.

Relaxation

Relaxation training (Mitchell 1988) is included in the daily activities of the course. The group explores the meaning of relaxation verses tension and how worry, fear, and anxiety can increase their state of tension which in turn can effect their fluency. They discuss ways in which they can adopt the relaxation techniques for use at home, school and social situations and its relevance to their own particular problem. The ability to use relaxation techniques successfully helps them in relation to their speech production as well as anxiety management.

Praise and Reinforcement

Adolescents often lack confidence and for an adolescent who stutters this can prove to be a serious problem. Increasing their self confidence involves teaching them how to give and receive encouragement and reinforcement in an appropriate manner. It is also important they learn to reevaluate themselves in a positive way appreciating their good qualities rather than being overwhelmed by their failures. This ability to reframe their experiences will enable them to reinforce both themselves and others which will lead to increased feelings of self worth and confidence.

Problem Solving

Teaching adolescents a framework for problem solving provides them with an effective means of dealing with the issues that confront them. How can I get my homework in on time? How can I cope better with teasing? are common examples. Discovering that there are many alternative ways of coping with a situation offers the adolescent choices as well as the opportunity to change their behaviour in a way that is more productive for both themselves and others.

Personal Construct Therapy

Working with adolescents on a two week intensive course using a combination of social skills training and fluency control techniques has been shown to be the more effective in the long term (Rustin & Purser 1983) than with either of these techniques on their own. However, there are some adolescents who still have considerable difficulty in transferring and maintaining their newly acquired skills. Exploring the personal construct systems of stuttering adolescents on an individual non-intensive basis had proved particularly useful in understanding the issues that might impede their progress towards fluency (Botterill & Cook 1987). In using the framework that personal construct therapy (Kelly 1955) provides we can view the adolescent as developing a system of personal constructs with which to make sense of the world. These are based on past experiences and help the individual to predict and therefore control to some extent the events that confront him or her. We would wish to prevent the adolescent developing a core role as a stutterer and a system of constructs that depends on this view of self.

It was decided therefore to allow individual time for each adolescent to explore his or her personal construct system using the *self characterization* and *repertory grid* techniques (Kelly 1955; Fransella 1972; Botterill & Cook 1987). These techniques examine the individual nature of each adolescent's view of themselves, their stuttering and other significant people in their life. They can give a unique insight into the difficulties one individual may encounter in becoming fluent, or indeed may help to illustrate the limited role the stutter plays in the life of another.

Self characterization

The adolescent is asked to write a character sketch of him or herself in the third person (Botterill & Cook 1987). They are encouraged to write a full account of themselves including their strengths and weaknesses. This is one way of eliciting some of the personal constructs they are using and allows them to talk about their prevailing concerns, which may range from their prowess on the football field to their lack of confidence talking to teachers. Further constructs can be elicited by asking the adolescent to think of various important people in their lives; e.g. mother, father, brother, best friend, teacher, and to find three things each of those people would say about them; e.g. they're untidy, they're funny, they're a good friend, etc. Other methods of eliciting constructs can also be employed and may need to be varied for the individuals concerned (Levy & Hayhow 1989).

Repertory Grid

The repertory grid contains a number of *constructs* that have been elicited in relation to a number of relevant *elements*. Since we are interested in interpersonal relationships, the elements should be significant people in the adolescent's life; e.g. mother, father, teacher, friend, etc. Once the elements and the constructs have been decided upon by the therapist and client, each element is rated with each construct in turn on a nine point scale, e.g. father may be rated as 8 on the construct *warm ....cold* (where 1 is the warmest and 9 the coldest).

The resulting data matrix can be analyzed using a computer programme (Higginbotham & Bannister 1983). Ultimately it becomes possible for the stutterers and the therapist to see hidden associations between elements and between constructs which assist in the planning of treatment. The whole process aims to help the adolescent and therapist work together to discover how the client sees him or her self and their current situation and, how they might proceed towards their desired goal.

Our experience over the last twelve months suggests that certain patterns are emerging. The adolescents seem broadly to fit into one of three groups.

Group One: The grids of these stutterers do not immediately show any particular areas of difficulty. These stutterers view of *self stuttering* and *self now* are very similar while the *ideal* self often leaves room for improvement but is not polarized. It would seem that their stuttering does not affect the way they see themselves or others in any significant way. Perhaps these individuals, whose stuttering is often mild, should reconstrue their need to *get rid of the stutter* as there seems little reason why they should invest the kind of effort necessary in becoming fluent.

Group Two: These stutterers grids pinpoint one or two constructs that actively prevent them from becoming fluent. For example, the student who sees *fluency* and talkative as being highly related to each other but in construing themselves would wish to be at the *quiet* end of the *talkative - quiet* construct. While this dilemma exists the stutterer cannot move towards fluency for fear of the consequences. Reconstruing of the various issues is required before changes can be made.

Group Three: For these clients the construct system revolves round the *fluent -stuttering* dimension. They tend to be more severe stutterers whose construct system is constricted to a point where they see themselves as separated from the rest of the world and people around them by their stuttering. These clients need to find new ways of construing themselves and others that will allow them to make socially useful predictions. These clients it seems will need to embark on major reconstruing before being able to risk fluency other than in the controlled and protected environment of the clinic.

Repertory grid technique enables us to make predictions regarding the adolescents ability to maintain fluency as well as helping them to have a better understanding of the changes they will need to make in order to transfer their fluency into the real world.

Those adolescents falling into groups 1 or 2 tend to be those for whom the two week intensive phase of the programme is particularly helpful - they may require some follow-up sessions to address the issues raised by their repertory grid, and to negotiate changes with family members, but therapy should not need to be long term. Therapy for group three individuals is aimed at helping them construe the changes that may need to take place before fluency becomes an option. They should be helped to understand (they are often relieved to find) that they really cannot be fluent until they have reconstrued themselves, as well as those around them and their stuttering in a way that will allow fluency. Their inability to transfer their fluency from the clinical setting can be better understood as an act of self preservation. This change in their understanding of their *failure* to achieve fluency will perhaps allow for the process of change to begin. Revised expectations should be concerned with the development and growth of their understanding of self, their perception of others and their interactions. The sense of guilt and failure that emanates from expectations of fluency having been finally removed.

Follow up Therapy

In order to transfer and maintain these new skills and changing attitudes, we need to call upon the family and perhaps the school to help. In the weeks immediately after the course the stutterer will begin to appreciate the difficulties involved in maintaining changes in behaviour. Members of the family should be involved in discussions with the adolescent in order to establish ways in which they can facilitate the process of change.

Family Session

The therapist should organise a session to which all members of the family are invited. The purpose of this meeting is to open up lines of communication that will enable them to negotiate issues more effectively. The first step in a family session (Rustin 1987a) would shape the way in which each family member should respond to the stuttering.

Paul aged 16, felt that his mother was **over helpful** and during the session it was negotiated that she would praise Paul's fluent speech 5 times a day but should only respond to his stuttering once per day (and not in front of others) by saying **Be Careful**. He wanted his sister, with whom he had a close relationship, to continue to **do nothing** as he found this very normal.

The second step in the session allows each individual to state a behaviour that they find irritating or difficult to deal with in the other members of the family.

Mrs. M. found it difficult to manage Matthew's aggressive behaviour towards his stuttering brother Mark. Matthew was asked how his mother should deal with this problem. He replied that she should spend more time with him. Mrs. M. had been devoting a significant amount of time to the stuttering brother at Matthew's expense. Fighting ceased following the negotiated settlement.

A contract is drawn up at the end of the session which records the agreements that have been negotiated. The family returns the following week to report on the success or failure of the contract and terms are re-negotiated where appropriate. Family sessions should be conducted on a weekly basis at home to monitor on-going issues and negotiate new contracts if necessary.

The therapist and adolescent continue to explore the process of change in regular, individual sessions. This may involve reconstruing situations involving communication difficulties or helping with other problem areas that may be undermining the student's self confidence and interfering with progress towards fluency.

S. had been making good progress in therapy following an intensive course. Family sessions had achieved an improvement in the family interactions and allowed the mother to take a passive role as far as the stuttering was concerned. Some months later a family session was organised as a result of a sudden increase in the stuttering and poor attendance by S. at the clinic. During the session it became clear that the problem was related to S's difficulty in managing his studying for his Advanced Level course. Previously an industrious student, S. was now opting out of any academic tasks. The family agreed to stop nagging, and S. agreed to a programme of behaviour modification to tackle his **work phobia**. This aimed at reducing his anxiety by structuring his studying into manageable units. Within a month his anxiety had decreased and he was able to cope with his academic workload. Following this episode he continued to make progress with his fluency.

At various stages it becomes necessary to help adolescents develop strategies for dealing with others beyond the family whose co-operation cannot be expected. Reconstruing stress and problem solving techniques can provide alternative ways of handling situations.

D. was fluent except with his mother whose **over protectiveness** was deeply frustrating to him. D. was the youngest son and the only sibling still at home. His mother, recently widowed, had great difficulty **letting go** of her **baby** and D. did not wish to upset her. D. was helped to understand his mother's behaviour and through this to help her adjust to his increasing independence in very small stages. The first step involved his telephoning her to say he would be five minutes late getting home, but only being slightly late. On the next occasion he was slightly earlier than usual - she was being helped to trust him and become more flexible in her expectations of him.

At the initial interview we advise people to expect to be in therapy for approximately two years. This would involve an intensive phase followed by weekly and then monthly sessions. The timetable adjusted according to the clients needs. We wish to engender the idea that therapy can be a long, hard road but that we are willing to support them all the way. We are not expecting instant results, remissions are taken for granted as are giant leaps. No-one need feel guilty if their disfluency overtakes them, it does not mean back to the beginning again as it has so often before.

In summary, this chapter addressed the particular problems of stuttering in adolescents. We discussed the growth of independence and the changing role of the family in the therapy process. The comprehensive approach to assessment and treatment was described in relation to an intensive course. A rational was provided for each component of the programme and clarified by brief examples. Finally the emergence of possible sub-groups through the use of the repertory grid technique was discussed in relation to therapy outcome.

Chapter 7

Therapy for Adolescents: Speech and Attitude Change

Hugo H. Gregory & Carolyn B. Gregory

In this chapter we will describe a system and philosophy of therapy for working with adolescents who stutter. Some of our observations will echo those discussed in Chapter 6. Basic approaches are grounded upon the way we understand the problem of stuttering. One of our clearest understandings is that, while we can delineate general principles of therapy and procedures stemming from these principles, there is no group of clients for whom therapy must be more individualized than for adolescents. Some of the individual characteristics which come up frequently in therapy will be noted in this chapter. Many others will be observed by clinicians as they relate to their clients and must be taken into consideration as the clinician uses a problem solving approach.

Evaluation

Though the focus of this chapter will be upon therapy, differential evaluation is an essential first step, and must be discussed briefly (See Chapter Four for detailed discussion of assessment). As in most clinical situations, evaluation includes a thorough case history, observations of speech and language, and the administration of certain tests. The young person usually comes with one or both parents. If there is a diagnostic team, the parents may be interviewed while the teenager is being evaluated. A developmental case history form facilitates the exploration of all important areas.

The importance of a sensitive client-centred listening approach with adolescents cannot be overemphasized. Adolescents with a stuttering problem usually have a long and frustrating history of being told what to do by various well-meaning adults, as well as experiencing teasing by their peers. Audiotape should be running during the interview in order to capture the full story as the youngster tells it, as well as for obtaining an extensive speech sample, but confidentiality is stressed.

Exploration should include:

1) how he/she sees the present problem;

2) why therapy is sought at the present time;

3) what has been done about the stuttering in the past;

4) what has seemed to be helpful;

5) earliest memories of life within the family as well as a history of the stuttering problem;

6) school experiences, including relationship with peers.

A thorough evaluation of the youngster's level of comfort and happiness in the home should probe sensitively such topics as relationships within the family, discipline style, ways of handling anger, history of marital unhappiness, divorce or separation, serious illnesses, important moves, etc. Hopefully, the youngsters react positively by seeing that the clinician wants to understand the uniqueness of their problems.

Video recording is utilized if available to sample a speech monologue, dialogue, time-pressed conversation, reading aloud, and making a telephone call for information. The client is not required to view it at this time.

If the young person expresses adequate motivation, a therapy plan is presented, including the basic duration (20-25 hours), tapering off to meetings once per week, or every two or three weeks and group sessions. At this point, the therapist will, with the youngster's consent, bring the parents into a discussion of the therapy plan. The general rule is that we are working with the young person and all plans to include others are worked out with him or her.

At the commencement of therapy a psychological developmental examination and pencil-and-paper personality and speech-attitude scales are performed (see Chapter 6). At this time a thorough analysis and frequency-count of the stuttering behaviour is drawn from the audio and video tapes.

Basic Principles Providing A Rationale for Therapy

The objective of therapy is the modification of unadaptive speech behavior and attitudes. In counterconditioning stuttering behavior, speech responses that are more adaptive and incompatible with stuttering are reinforced in the presence of stimuli that previously led to stuttering (e.g. a word or a situation). The more adaptive response may be either modified stuttering or a fluency enhancing procedure such as an easier onset. A desensitization approach is used in that responses are changed first in the presence of stimuli that have a history of evoking minimal stuttering and associated negative emotion (easier situations), and then in situations that have been associated with increased stuttering (more difficult situations). One of the clinician's most important functions is to arrange for change to occur in graduated steps from shorter units of speech to longer ones, from less meaningful to more meaningful content, and from less stressful to more stressful situations. By using a hierarchy in this way overt speech responses, the significance of stimulus conditions and covert emotional responses are being worked with simultaneously. Thus, generalization and transfer are occurring from the beginning of therapy.

Attitudes (feelings and thoughts) are dealt with by being open and making an honest effort to understand how the young person perceives the problem, by providing information about stuttering and the process of therapy, by exploring reactions to the therapeutic process - especially as they relate to parental expectation, practice at home, and transfer into real situations at school or in social life.

Self-monitoring, self-evaluation and self-reinforcement are emphasized from the beginning of therapy. This is important during the initial stages of therapy, but very crucial during the transfer and maintenance or follow through period. When there is objection to *monitoring* speech, it is helpful to point out that this is a superior skill used by trained speakers (not just stutterers) and that it can be a lot more dependable than *just winging it.*

Another insight for the youngster to experience is, *you have always tried to hide your stuttering, and pay as little attention to it as you could. You have tried hard not to think about talking. It's only natural for it to seem strange now to pay close attention to the way you talk. You are learning the skills of above-average speech when you monitor.*

Combining the Stutter-More-Fluently and the Speak-More-Fluently Models

Clinicians such as Bloodstein (1958), Johnson (1967), Sheehan (1970) and Van Riper (1973), who based their work on a stutter-more-fluently frame of reference, stressed that stutterers with a confirmed problem should not be given some method to stop stuttering and readily produce fluency, but that they should learn to attend to their stuttering, monitor it, and then gradually modify their speech by thinking of and seeing how they can stutter more easily

(Gregory 1979). In this way, stutterers are not avoiding stuttering as much because they are studying and modifying it. Youngsters are attracted by the idea of facing up to fear, doing the thing that is hard, taking a scientific approach to studying their stuttering. Reduced fear and avoidance results in increased fluency.

Replacing stuttering with various forms of fluent speech has been taught by several contributors such as Ryan (1974, 1979), Wingate (1976), Perkins (1979), and Webster (1979). Fluency initially obtained by using such procedures as delayed auditory feedback or instruction in the modification of various parameters of speech such as rate, voice onset, air-voice flow, and blending, is shaped to accomplish speech that is considered normally fluent (Gregory 1979). We have never had a teenager yet who objected to this aspect of therapy. They love working on fluency.

In working with stutterers who have a confirmed problem, there are inadequacies in both a therapy that focuses only on *stuttering more fluently* - i.e. the reduction of inhibition and avoidance by analyzing and modifying stuttering, and a therapy that focuses on *speaking more fluently* - i.e. fluency shaping with little or no attention to monitoring and changing moments of stuttering. A combination of the two models appears to be best in terms of reducing the degree of regression, or put another way, of helping the person to cope with the variations in fluency that will occur after therapy. It should be emphasized from the beginning that stuttering varied before therapy and it will after therapy, and that a period of follow-up is essential for the person to adjust to the changes that have taken place.

The sequence of procedures that we shall describe with reference to speech and attitudinal changes are viewed as combining the two models (Gregory 1968, 1979, 1986; Gregory & Gregory 1984). Confirmed stutterers study and monitor unadaptive stuttering behavior and other characteristics such as rapid rate, tense glottal attack, erratic prosody, etc. Then they learn to change their speech, easing the tension, slowing a repetition, reducing a prolongation, etc. To this point, monitoring and gradually changing, but not eliminating stuttering is emphasized. Finally, through relaxed speech onsets, smooth movements between sounds, syllables, and words, phrasing with attention to proper pausing between phrases, and improved speech skills (variation of rate, loudness, and inflection), behavior that is counter to stuttering and conducive to more fluent speech is learned.

In combining the two models there is a paradox of which stutterers and their clinicians should be aware. Analysis and acceptance of stuttering as a part of therapy contradicts

105

building fluency and vice-versa. This understanding is a part of the attitudinal aspect of therapy, of understanding the tricky nature of stuttering, and perhaps even the tricky nature of therapy.

A major advantage of combining the two approaches is that stutterers learn to cope with moments of stuttering, resulting in reduced sensitivity about stuttering and diminished fear of regression or relapse when stuttering occurs. They also increase skills appropriate for normal fluency. Both the unadaptive speech habits and the learned negative emotional responses are counterconditioned.

The Usual Sequence of Procedures

We will describe procedures by objective and with reference to speech changes and attitudinal considerations.

Objective: Identifying Speech Characteristics

Speech. The client and the clinician listen to short segments of the client's tape recorded connected speech, stopping the recorder to discuss certain characteristics such as **tense repetitions of the first syllable, excess escape of air followed by increased tension and pushing through the block, rapid rate**, etc. As the client adjusts to this exercise, viewing a video playback may be added. It is important to mention that viewing oneself on video is always disquieting at first. The clinician and the client cooperate in making a list describing characteristics of the stutterer's speech.

Attitude. It is stressed that this first step in therapy takes considerable courage; that it is hard to do, but essential. The clinician provides support by pointing out what is being learned and by reinforcing the client's observations. The client should understand that they are beginning to study their stuttering where in the past they have always focused on hiding and avoiding it. In this respect the more avoidant and interiorized the stuttering has been, the more resistant is the client to feeling and experiencing it. While the teens are a time of confrontation, when handled sensitively by the therapist, this phase is tolerated well.

Objective: Negative Practice (2 Degrees of Tension)

Speech. Working first with some of the words drawn from the stutterer's own speech, the client is encouraged to imitate his or her stuttering to do on a more voluntary basis what is involuntary when they actually stutter. When the stutterer imitates a block, they often observe that they are *easing it up*. At first we say, *Try to do it just the way you ordinarily do*. During the next session, we may introduce negative practice on lists containing a random selection of words. Sometimes the negative practice becomes real stuttering. This may be frightening, but it is what we want to happen. It gives the client a real laboratory in which to experience stuttering in a safe environment and monitor carefully. Next, 50% reduction is introduced in which the person imitates stuttering as closely as possible, then repeats the word reducing tension by about 50%.

Attitude. The young person is reinforced for *putting stuttering out on the table*, for making it the object of study. For the first time, someone has smiled and clapped his hands for a stutter well-produced! This is healing. As a result of this experimentation during negative practice, the person begins to realize that he or she can change aspects of their speech. In fact, most begin to experience less stuttering and more fluency. We discuss with the stutterer the avoidance and inhibition which has been relieved by this exercise. We describe our hypothesis where, as a child, either normal or somewhat atypical disfluency may have been avoided. Later it was stuttering that was being inhibited, resulting in the present way of talking. We emphasize that an important first step is to monitor the sensations associated with the tension of stuttering.

Objective: More Easy Relaxed Approach, Smooth Movement (ERA-SM)

Speech. Stuttering and other maladaptive aspects of speaking have been studied in a variety of ways. ERA-SM is a procedure for continuing the process of speech modification in which the client does the following:

(l) In practising words, the initial consonant vowel (CV) or vowel consonant (VC) combination is produced with a more relaxed, smooth movement that is slightly slower than usual. The remainder of the word beyond the initial CV or VC transition is produced at the normal rate and with normal inflection, but with consciously smoother movement and relaxed articulators.

(2) In the case of phrases, ERA-SM is emphasized on the first CV or VC combination of the first word, then the remainder of the word and subsequent words in the phrase are blended together. In connected discourse, phrasing is emphasized using ERA-SM

at the beginning of each phrase. Stutterers show a tendency to take anticipatory positions, such as closing the lips for /p/, rather than thinking of the /p/ and the following vowel as a smooth movement. This is practised on words and phrases. A key point is that the clinician asks the client to contrast ERA-SM with degrees of tension purposely introduced as in negative practice.

Attitude. The client is helped to see that they are counterconditioning the maladaptive stuttering (excess tension and fragmentation of speech flow) by practising more adaptive behaviour (more easy-relaxed-smooth movements). Analogies are made to modifying other motor activities such as the swing of a golf club or a tennis racket. When changing a habit, the activity has to be slowed up, etc.

Adjusting to change is discussed. Stutterers and individuals with other speech and voice problems find it difficult to accept change. Adolescents are more aware of their change than adults and project this awareness on to their listeners. As Sheehan (1970) said, the familiar will feel *right* even though it is objectively *wrong*, whereas the unfamiliar will feel *wrong* even though objectively it is correct. Having the youngster listen to audiotapes and view videotapes has been found valuable. It takes time to accept change.

Finally, continuing negative practice and contrasting this with ERA-SM continues the process of reducing sensitivity about stuttering and builds confidence in the ability to make a choice.

Objective: Resisting Time Pressure (Delayed Response)

Speech. Time pressure is a natural aspect of communication. When a person is speaking, they feel that another is awaiting a turn. (See Chapters 5 & 6 for detailed discussion on turntaking.) Stutterers feel this, but they also experience stress from knowing that there will be difficulty initiating speech. Once the client gains confidence in being able to initiate speech better, work can be done on counterconditioning time pressure. Using a word list (now also using ERA-SM), clients count to one or two in their minds before saying a word. They make a point of varying the pause between phrases. When answering questions, especially those where they are asked to repeat what they have just said, they practice delaying.

Attitude. The client's fear of silence or of holding up the person to whom they are talking when stuttering is counterconditioned. We point out that effective communication is not rushed. The person who stutters should say to him or herself: *I can hold myself up some,*

I can resist the pressure I feel from others. Young people, especially teenagers, have exaggerated ideas of how fast their peers speak, and of how important it is not to be viewed as *different*. Resisting time pressure is a skill they enjoy using with their parents, and one they can take pride in using to show courage in changing patterns of speech in spite of peer pressure.

Objective: Voluntary Disfluency

Speech. This is to be distinguished from voluntary stuttering (emitting a stutter like behavior voluntarily in conversation) and negative practice. After the stutterer's speech has shown considerable improvement and as they are beginning to realize that they have more options, we teach the use of some voluntary disfluency like that emitted by non-stuttering speakers, and of course, by stutterers too as part of the normal production of speech. Word repetition such as *I, I* or *in, in*, phrase repetition such as *I want, I want, it's, it's* and interjections such as *well uh* are some examples.

Attitude. When stutterers' fluency increases, they need to deal with their hypersensitivity about disfluency or stuttering, an attitude that is easily understood. This attitude has developed from childhood as the youngster attempted to speak more fluently and hide disfluency and stuttering. Teenage stutterers will want perfect fluency. They will desire *superfluency*. Voluntary disfluency helps to countercondition this tendency.

The client should say, *I am gaining more flexibility and confidence in my speech. I can even be disfluent on purpose. This helps to reduce my sensitivity about disfluency or stuttering*.

Objective: Increasing Flexibility

Speech. This refers to learning to vary rate, loudness, inflection, pause time, etc. From the beginning of therapy, we tell stutterers that the techniques we are teaching them, such as phrasing, are good habits of speaking. Throughout the process of speech change, we attempt to keep the client's normal prosody intact. At this point we give instruction in varying phrase length and show the youngster how variation in the parameters of rate, loudness, and inflection are characteristics of skilful speakers. We do this in the context of knowing that some stuttering may need to be dealt with and that some voluntary disfluency will be beneficial.

Attitude: The attitude that we aim for is that even though a person may be coping with the occurrence of some minimal stuttering, they can still be a good speaker. But, of course, if the person is successful with the whole therapeutic strategy he or she will communicate better and better, stutter less and less and be steadily more comfortable and effective as a speaker.

The Hierarchy

As discussed earlier, for speech modification to be successful, change should be made first in easier situations and then gradually in more difficult ones. We have described how this principle is being practised as we go from shorter to longer and from less meaningful to more meaningful utterances. At this point, although we are focusing on transfer from easier to more difficult speaking situations, the reader can see that utterance length and propositionality is not completely separated from this. All three - length, propositionality and situation - are systematically integrated. The therapist works with the teenager to work out the hierarchy.

Here is an example of from less difficult to more difficult:

1 Clinic room with clinician
2 Clinic room, with another client
3 Lounge with another client
4 Clinic room with a friend
5 Lounge with a friend
6 Walking around the building with the clinician
7 Clinic room or lounge with his mother
8 Making a telephone call to inquire about a product
9 Telephoning to friend
10 Short conversation with mother or father
11 Short conversation with a friend at school

This is enough to describe the concept. We say to clients as we say to therapists reading this chapter, *Hierarchies really work!* Careful construction and revision of the hierarchy, and finally execution of it, is crucial to the success of therapy. Of course, the therapist intervenes to organize the steps in ways that are more likely to lead to success. It should be self-evident that in constructing a hierarchy, psychological comfort with the family members chosen to work with the young stutterer is essential.

Group process

Adolescents are at a stage in life during which they are extremely sensitive to being singled out as a youngster with a unique problem. Their distress is immediately lowered when they can see and share experiences with someone else who is *in the same boat*. Even during the intensive individual phase of therapy, it is helpful for the young stutterer to meet another who may be doing similar assignments, or having similar feelings about not sounding *natural*, or resisting time pressure. At the time therapy can safely be reduced to twice monthly or monthly, a teenage group is an ideal setting in which the youngsters can bring back and share their *horror stories*, laugh over them, and inspire each other to continue courageously. Being successful at stuttering therapy takes courage. It might be added that for some young people, a therapy group may be the first experience with caring friends with whom to practice telephone calls and so on.

Supplementary Techniques

We have adapted Van Riper's (1973) **cancellation and pull-out procedures**. In conjunction with the teaching of negative practice, the client is shown how to modify stuttering as it occurs, i.e. pull-out of the block. Thus, the person is asked to imitate their stuttering carefully, first at *full tension*, then at 50% reduction, and finally (using a slight prolongation), to pull-out. This ability is reemphasized in the latter stages of therapy. Cancellation is taught by having the stutterer stop immediately when he or she senses a block and make an altered, more easy-relaxed approach to the word. Since our easy-relaxed-approach smooth-movement (ERA-SM) method is based so firmly in phrasing (i.e. smooth co-articulation of the phrase), the person may also go back to the beginning of the phrase unit when he or she senses a block. Of course, they must begin the phrase with an easy relaxed onset and make the movement through the phrase smoothly. In these ways, the experience (or the behavior) of blocking is cancelled.

Delayed Auditory Feedback (DAF) has been found useful with those cases who find it difficult to modify their speech following the clinician's model. DAF may be helpful when a youngster has a rapid rate with many small stutters. It may be used if the speech is characterized by elements of cluttering. DAF is especially helpful when specific control of rate and prosody are desired.

Since tension that interferes with the smooth flow of speech is seen as a major part of the problem, we incorporate the use of progressive and differential muscle relaxation as described by Jacobson (1938). The person is encouraged to reduce bodily tension while modifying speech. People who stutter agree readily that tension is involved in stuttering and see the relationship between reducing general bodily tension and modifying tension in the speech mechanism. We do not say, *be relaxed*, but rather we teach the person to reduce bodily tension.

Follow-up

Stuttering therapy is not short term. After a core period of therapy of three to six months, a follow through programme of 12-18 months is required. Just as non-stutterers have varying feelings of confidence about certain life situations, stutterers need to realize that they will continue to experience challenging situations that will require additional analysis and planning. Returning to the clinic for review sessions must be viewed as a positive thing to do. Most clinics and private practitioners now provide what we term a continuation programme, often called maintenance.

Individual Psychological Factors

As has been emphasized earlier, a basic characteristic of therapy with a teenager is a personal rapport that encourages a deep sharing of life outside the therapy room. This sharing includes such things as successes and failures with specific speech tasks, and additionally, very personal joys and disappointments, and sometimes the depths of sadness, anger, or shame.

Even within the intact, sound family background which has existed without serious trauma from the earliest memory of the client, there are still broad differences in parenting styles, discipline, higher or lower expectations, rigidity or relaxation of routines, speed of talking, competitiveness, relationship with siblings, etc. It is essential to know the home in order to

112

choose appropriate speech assignments to be carried out realistically. (See Chapters 1, 5 & 6 for more detail on family assessment.)

There are wide differences in the degree of shame experienced in stuttering, and the willingness to share this with a parent, sibling or friend. Early in therapy, the youngster is encouraged to choose one person with whom to share therapy activities at first, and then to build on this by being more open about the stuttering problem and the therapy process with others.

The introversion-extroversion style of the client is an important factor which can be modified only slightly. More sensitive and withdrawn young people can learn to accept and value their own nature, but must be drawn more carefully through a hierarchy. They must be encouraged to join a club or after-school activity, to develop an interest which requires telephoning or library research, to seek a job in which talking will be required. If you cannot entice a youngster to develop some useful speaking situations, therapy will be in trouble. Often, these more withdrawn teenagers, often quite intelligent, are less motivated to make speech changes and choose to relate to computers or laboratory equipment instead of humans. In this connection, social skills training (Rustin & Kuhr 1989) may be an essential aspect of therapy.

Anger, sometimes unreasonable rage, at being teased by peers, insensitive teachers or other adults must be handled by extensive talking through, and sometimes by a simultaneous psychological referral. This anger may have resulted in excessive shame, strong situational avoidances, and perhaps very severe blocking requiring the building of creative hierarchies and development of humour and insight - tasks that may tax the wits of the therapist.

We have all known youngsters from less-than-ideal circumstances. This brings to mind the tall sullen high-school football star with a long silent shameful-looking block (20-30 seconds) who had allergies, felt miserable most of the time, and had been labelled the black sheep of the family. His anger flared instantly, and it was known at school that he would punch anyone who even smiled at his stuttering. He had high motivation and developed considerable pride in knocking on doors and seeking jobs on his own. His father helped by purchasing a truck, and helping him to start a business. The inappropriate violence was brought under control with the help of a psychologist and counselling for the family.

Another challenging boy (child of a former rejected spouse) lived with his mother and stepfather and three very small step sisters. This family had a style of ignoring the teenager, talking fast, interrupting one another and appearing to be totally absorbed in the activities of the little girls. The parents chose not to notice any of the speech changes the boy attempted to make and accused him of not practising, etc. All the time, he was making important progress in school. He was removed from therapy by the righteous parents who insisted he was unmotivated.

Another child of divorce got along very poorly with his mother (with whom he lived) and did not feel that his attractive new stepmother was really interested in helping him. He was not strong physically, had suffered much teasing from a few bullies in school, and seemed to attract teasing by his sensitivity. This case required time for the boy to adjust to his father's new partner, for his trust in his stepmother to take place, for him to accept the necessity for self-monitoring his speech. The gradual letting go of the sensitivity was a joy to watch from the clinician's point of view - he finally squared off with the bullies from his position in authority in a record store.

These case histories point up the very individual solution to each problem of stuttering, and the challenge of being a specialist in stuttering disorders. Clinicians who are especially interested in working with adolescents should have knowledge of the literature on the psychodynamics of adolescence and should participate in continuing education opportunities to up-date their understanding of developments in this area.

Summary

Therapy for adolescent stutterers has been described with reference to several basic principles that provide a rationale for the decision making process involved. The description of a sequence of activities with reference to speech and attitude change is based on our experience of combining the *stutter-more-fluently* and the *speak-more-fluently* models. We emphasize that while there are commonalities in the approach to therapy, each client must be treated as an individual. Thus, we have delineated optional supplementary techniques that can be utilized and given examples of more general psychological problems that may need attention.

REFERENCES

Adams, M. 1980. The young stutterer: diagnosis, treatments, and assessment of progress. *Seminars in Speech, Language, and Hearing* 4, 289-299.

Adams, M., Freeman, F. & Conture, E. 1984. Laryngeal dynamics of stutterers. In: R. Curlee & W. Perkins (Eds.), *Nature and Treatment of Stuttering: New Directions*. San Diego, California: College-Hill Press.

Ainsworth, S. 1988. *If Your Child Stutters* (3rd edition). Memphis: Speech Foundation of America.

American Speech-Language-Hearing Association 1984. Guidelines for caseload size for speech-language services in the schools. *ASHA* 26, 53-58.

Anders, T.F. 1980. The development of sleep patterns and sleep disturbances from infancy through adolescence. In: B. Camp (Ed.), *Advances in Behavioral Paediatrics (Vol 2)*. Greenwich,Conn: JAI Press.

Andrews, J. & Andrews, M. 1983. A family approach to the treatment of speech-language disorders. In: M. Edwards (Ed.), *Proceedings of the XIX Congress of the IALP*. London: The College of Speech Therapists.

Andrews J. & Andrews, M. 1989. *Family systems and treatment: understanding the systemic perspective*. Short Course presented at the ASHA Convention, St. Louis.

Andrews, G., Craig, A., Feyer, A.M., Hoddinott, S., Howie, P. & Neilson, M. 1983 Stuttering: a review of research findings and theories circa 1982. *Journal of Speech and Hearing Disorders* 48, 226-246.

Andrews, G. & Harris, M. 1964. *The Syndrome of Stuttering*. London: Spastics Society.

Andronico, M, & Blake, I 1971. The application of filial therapy to young children with stuttering problems. *Journal of Speech and Hearing Disorders* 36, 377-381.

Atal, B., Chang, J., Mathews, M., & Tukey, J. 1978. Inversion of articulatory-to-acoustic transformation in the vocal tract by computer-sorting technique. *Journal of Acoustical Society of America* 63, 1535-1555.

Beech, H. & Fransella, F. 1968. *Research and Experiment in Stuttering*. Oxford: Pergamon Press.

Bernstein-Ratner, N., & Costa, S.C. 1987. Effects of gradual increases in sentence length and complexity on children's dysfluency. *Journal of Speech and Hearing Disorders* 52, 278-287.

Blakeley, R. 1980. *Screening Test for Developmental Apraxia of Speech*. Tigard, OR: C.C. Publications.

Bloodstein, O. 1958 Stuttering as an anticipatory struggle reaction. In J. Eisenson (Ed.), *Stuttering: A Symposium*. New York: Harper and Row.

Bloodstein, O. 1987. *A Handbook on Stuttering* (4th edition). Chicago: The National Easter Seal Society.

Borden, G., Kim, D. & K. Spiegler 1987. Acoustics of stop consonant-vowel relationships during fluent and stuttered utterances. *Journal of Fluency Disorders* 12, 175-184.

Botterill, W. & Cook, F. 1987. Personal construct theory and the treatment of adolescent dysfluency. In L. Rustin, H. Purser and D. Rowley (Eds.), *Progress in the Treatment of Fluency Disorders*. London: Whurr.

Brutten, E.J. & Shoemaker, D.J. 1967. *The Modification of Stuttering*. Prentice-Hall: Engelwood Cliffs, NJ.

Button, L. 1980. *Developmental Group Work with Adolescents*. London: Hodder & Stoughton

Byrd, K. & Cooper, E. 1989. Apraxic speech characteristics in stuttering, developmentally apraxic, and normal speaking children. *Journal of Fluency Disorders* 14, 215-229.

Byrne, R. 1984. *Let's Talk About Stammering*. London: Unwin Paperbacks.

Caruso, A., Abbs, J., & Gracco, V. 1988. Kinematic analysis of multiple movement coordination during speech in stutterers. *Brain* 111, 439-455.

Caruso, A., Conture, E. & Colton, R. 1988. Selected temporal patterns of coordination associated with stuttering in children. *Journal of Fluency Disorders* 13, 57-82.

Cath, S., Gurwitt, A. & Gunsberg, L. 1989. Fathers and Their Families. Hillsdale, NJ: The Analytic Press.

Clarke-Stewart, A. 1977. *The father's impact on mother and child*. Paper presented at the biennial meeting of the Society for Research in Child Development, New Orleans, March.

Colton, R. & Conture, E. 1990. Problems and pitfalls in the use of electroglottography. *Journal of Voice* 4, 10-24.

Conture, E. 1982. Youngsters who stutter: diagnosis, parent counselling and referral. *Journal of Developmental Behavioral Paediatrics* 3, 163-169.

Conture, E. 1987. Studying young stutterers' speech production: a procedural challenge. In H. Peters & W. Hulstijn (Eds.), *Speech Motor Dynamics in Stuttering*. New York: Springer-Verlag.

Conture, E. 1990a. Childhood stuttering: what is it and who does it? In J. A. Cooper (Ed.), *Research Needs in Stuttering: Roadblocks and Future Directions*. ASHA Reports 18.

Conture, E. 1990b. *Stuttering* (2nd ed.). Englewood Cliffs, NJ: Prentice-Hall.

Conture, E., Colton, R., & Gleason, J. 1988. Selected temporal aspects of coordination during young stutterers fluent speech. *Journal of Speech Hearing Research* 31, 640-653.

Conture, E. & Fraser, J. (Eds.) 1989. *Stuttering and Your Child: Questions and Answers*. Memphis, TN: Speech Foundation of America.

Conture, E., Rothenberg, M. & Molitor, R. 1986. Electroglottographic observations of young stutterers' fluency. *Journal of Speech and Hearing Research* 29, 384-393.

Conture, E. & Caruso, A. 1987. Assessment and diagnosis of childhood dysfluency. In L. Rustin, H. Purser and D. Rowley (Eds.), *Progress in the Treatment of Fluency Disorders*. London: Taylor and Francis.

Cooper, E. & Cooper, C. 1985. *Personalized Fluency Control Therapy. Revised.*

Costello, J. M. 1983. Current behavioural treatment for children. In: D. Prins & R. Ingham (Eds.), *Treatment of Stuttering in Early Childhood*. San Diago: College-Hill Press.

Culp, D. 1984. The preschool fluency development program: assessment and treatment. In: M. Peins (Ed.), *Contemporary Approaches in Stuttering Therapy*. Boston: Little Brown.

Dunn, L. M. & Dunn, L. M. 1982. *British Picture Vocabulary Scale*. Windsor: NFER-Nelson.

Enger, N., Hood, S., & Shulman, B. 1988. Language and fluency variables in the conversational speech of linguistically advanced preschool and school-aged children. *Journal of Fluency Disorders* 13, 173-198.

Feldman, R. 1976. Self-disclosure in parents of stuttering children. *Journal of Communication Disorders* 9, 227-234.

Flavell, J. 1974. The development of inferences about others. In: T. Mischel (Ed.), *Understanding Other Persons*. Oxford: Blackwell, Basil & Mott.

Fletcher, S. 1972. Time-by-count measurement of diadochokinetic syllable rate. *Journal of Speech and Hearing Research* 15, 763-77.

Fransella, F. 1972. *Personal Change and Reconstruction: Research on a Treatment for Stuttering*. London: Academic Press.

Gelman, R. 1969. Conservation acquisition: a problem of learning to attend to relevant attributes. *Journal of Experimental Child Psychology* 7, 167-187.

Gelman, R. & Baillargeon, R. 1983. A review of some Piagetian concepts. In: P.H. Mussen (Ed.), *Carmichael's Manual of Child Psychology (Vol III)*. New York: Wiley.

Goodstein, L. 1956. MMPI profiles of stutterers' parents: a follow-up study. *Journal of Speech and Hearing Disorders* 21, 430-435.

Gregory, H. 1968. Applications of learning theory concepts in the treatment of stuttering. In: H. Gregory (Ed.), *Learning Theory and Stuttering Therapy*. Evanston, Ill: Northwestern University Press.

Gregory, H. 1979. Controversial issues: statement and review of the issues. In: H. Gregory (Ed.), *Controversies About Stuttering Therapy*. Baltimore: University Park Press.

Gregory, H. 1984. Prevention of stuttering: management of early stages. In: R. Curlee & W. Perkins (Eds.), *Nature and Treatment of Stuttering: New Directions*. San Diego: College-Hill Press.

Gregory, H. 1986a. Stuttering: a contemporary perspective. *Folia Phoniatrica* 38, 89-120.

Gregory, H. 1986b. Environmental manipulation and family counselling. In: G. Shames & H. Rubin (Eds.), *Stuttering: Then and Now*. Columbus, OH: Charles E. Merrill Publishing Company.

Gregory, H. & Gregory, C. 1984. *Combining the stutter-more-fluently and the speak-more-fluently approaches in stuttering therapy*. Short Course, ASHA

Convention, San Francisco.

Gregory, H. & Hill, D. 1980. Stuttering therapy for children. *Seminars in Speech, Language, and Hearing* 4, 351-364.

Gregory, H. & Hill, D. 1984. Stuttering therapy for children. In: W. Perkins (Ed.), *Stuttering Disorders*. New York: Thieme-Stratton.

Grossman, D. 1952. A study of the parents of stuttering and non-stuttering children using the Minnesota Multiphasic Personality Inventory and the Minnesota Scale of Parents' Opinions. *Speech Monograph* 19, 193-194.

Hayhow, R. 1983. The assessment of stuttering and the evaluation of treatment. In P. Dalton (ed.), *Approaches to the Treatment of Stuttering.* London: Croom Helm.

Hayhow, R. & Levy, C. 1989. *Working With Stuttering.* Windsor: Winslow Press.

Haynes, W. & Hood, S. 1978. Disfluency changes in children as a function of the systematic modification of linguistic complexity. *Journal of Community Disorders* 11, 79-93.

Helps, R. & Dalton, P. 1979. The effectiveness of an intensive group therapy programme for adult stammerers. *The British Journal of Disorders of Communication* 14, 17-30.

Hersov, L.A. 1977 School refusal. In: M. Rutter & L. Hersov (Eds.), *Child Psychiatry: Modern Approaches.* Oxford: Blackwell.

Higginbotham, P & Bannister, D. 1983. *The GAB computer programme for the analysis of repertory grid data.* Department of Psychology, University of Leeds, UK.

Irwin, A. 1988. *Stammering in Young Children.* Northampton: Thorsons Publishing.

Jacobson, E. I938. *Progressive Relaxation.* Chicago: University of Chicago Press.

Johnson, W. 1942. A study of the onset and development of stuttering. *Journal of Speech Disorders* 7, 251-257.

Johnson, W. I967 Stuttering. In: W. Johnson & D. Moeller (Eds.), *Speech Handicapped School Children.* New York: Harper and Row.

Johnson, W., Boehmler, R., Dahlstrom, W., Darley, F., Goodstein, L., Kools, S., Neeley, J., Prather, W., Sherman, D., Thurman, C., Trotter, W. & Williams, D. 1959. *The Onset of Stuttering.* Minneapolis: University of Minnesota Press.

Kasprisin-Burrelli, A., Egolf, D., & Shames, G. 1972. A comparison of parental verbal behavior with stuttering and nonstuttering children. *Journal of Communication Disorders* 5, 335-346.

Kelly, G.A. 1955. *The Psychology of Personal Constructs, Vol I.* New York: Norton.

Kidd, K. 1983. Recent progress on the genetics of stuttering. In: C. Ludlow & J. Cooper (Eds.), New York: Academic Press.

Kilburg, G., Lubker, B., Peins, M., St. Louis, K., Scherz, J., Sparks, S., & Cole, L. 1988. Prevention of communication disorders. *ASHA* 30, 90.

Kinstler, D. 1961. Covert and overt maternal rejection in stuttering. *Journal of Speech and Hearing Disorders* 26, 145-155.

Kuo, Z. 1976. *The Dynamics of Behavior Development: An Epigenetic View.* New

References

York: Random House.

Lafollette, A. 1956. Parental environment of stuttering children. *Journal of Speech and Hearing Disorders* 21, 202-207.

Lamb, M. 1977. Father-child and mother-child interaction in the first year of life. *Child Development* 48, 167-181.

Louko, L., Edwards, M., & Conture, E. In press. Phonological characteristics of young stutterers and their normally fluent peers: Preliminary observations. *Journal of Fluency Disorders.*

Luterman, D. 1984. *Counselling the Communicatively Disordered and their Families.* Boston, MA: Little Brown.

Mallard, A. 1989. A British-American co-operative effort in stuttering therapy: three year progress report. *Bulletin of the College of Speech Therapists* 477 (July), 2-4.

Mallard, A. & Westbrook, J. 1988. Variables affecting stuttering therapy in school settings. *Language, Speech, and Hearing Services in Schools* 19, 362-370.

Martin, R. & Lindamood, L. 1986. Stuttering and spontaneous recovery: implications for the speech pathologist. *Language, Speech, and Hearing Services in the Schools* 17, 207-218.

Masangkay, Z., McCluskey, K., McIntyre, C., Sims-Knight, J., Vaughn, B., & Flavell, J. 1974. The early development of inferences about the visual percepts of others. *Child Development* 45, 357-366.

Merits-Patterson, R. & Reed, C. 1981. Disfluencies in the speech of language-delayed children. *Journal of Speech and Hearing Research* 46, 55-58.

Meyers, S. 1986. Qualitative and quantitative differences and patterns of variability in disfluencies emitted by preschool stutterers and nonstutterers during dyadic conversations. *Journal of Fluency Disorders* 11, 293.

Meyers, S. 1989. Nonfluencies of preschool stutterers and conversational partners: observing reciprocal relationships. *Journal of Speech and Hearing Disorders* 54, 106-112.

Meyers, S. 1990. Verbal behaviors of preschool stutterers and conversational partners: Observing reciprocal relationships. In review.

Meyers, S. & Freeman, F. 1985a. Are mothers of stutterers different? An investigation of social-communicative interactions. *Journal of Fluency Disorders* 10, 193-209.

Meyers, S & Freeman, S. 1985b. Interruptions as a variable in stuttering and disfluency. *Journal of Speech and Hearing Research* 28, 428-435.

Meyers, S. & Freeman, F. 1985c. Mother and child speech rates as a variable in stuttering and disfluency. *Journal of Speech and Hearing Research* 28, 436-444.

Miller, J. 1981. *Assessing language production in children: experimental procedures.* Austin, TX: Pro-Ed.

Miller, J. & Chapman, R. 1986. *Systematic Analysis of Language Transcripts.* Madison: Language Analysis Laboratory, University of Wisconsin.

Mitchell, L. 1988. *Simple Relaxation: The Physiological Method for Easing Tension.*

119

London: John Murray.

Mordecai, D. 1979. An investigation of the communicative styles of mothers and fathers of stuttering versus nonstuttering preschool children. *Dissertation Abstracts International* 40, 4759-B.

Moore, W.H. and Boberg, E. 1987. Hemispheric processing and stuttering. In: L. Rustin, H. Purser & D. Rowley (Eds.), *Progress in the Treatment of Fluency Disorders*. Taylor & Francis: London.

Moses, K. 1985. Dynamic intervention with families. In: *Hearing-Impaired Children and Youth with Developmental Disabilities: An Interdisciplinary Foundation for Service*. Washington, D.C.: Gallaudet College Press.

Mowrer, D. 1972. Accountability and speech therapy in the public schools. *ASHA* 14, 111-115.

Newman, L. & Smit, A. 1989. Some effects of variations in response time latency on speech rate, interruptions, and fluency in children's speech. *Journal of Speech and Hearing Research* 32, 635-644.

Nelson, L. 1982. Language formulation related to disfluency and stuttering. In: *Stuttering Therapy: Prevention and Intervention with Children*. Memphis: Speech Foundation of America.

Orton, S. & Travis, L. 1929. Studies in stuttering IV: Studies of action currents in stutterers. *Archives in Neurology and Psychiatry* 21, 61-68.

Perkins, W. 1973. Replacement of stuttering with normal speech: 1. rationale. *Journal of Speech and Hearing Disorders* 38, 283-294.

Perkins, W. 1979 From psychoanalysis to discoordination. In H. Gregory (Ed.), *Controversies About Stuttering Therapy*. Baltimore: University Park Press.

Perkins, W. 1980. Strategies in stuttering therapy. *Seminars in Speech, Language, and Hearing* I, 9-11.

Peters, J., Romine, J. & Dykman, R. 1975. A special neurological examination of children with learning disabilities. *Developmental Medicine and Child Neurology* 17, 63-78.

Piaget, J. 1926. *The Language and Thought of the Child*. New York: Harcourt Brace.

Pindzola, R. 1986. Acoustic evidence of aberrant velocities in stutterers' fluent speech. *Perceptual and Motor Skills* 62, 399-405.

Prins, D. 1983. Continuity fragmentation and tension: hypothesis applied to evaluation and intervention with preschool dysfluent children. In: D. Prins & R. Ingham (Eds.), *Treatment of Stuttering in Early Childhood*. San Diago: College Hill Press.

Quarrington, B. 1966. The young stuttering child: a problem in management and research. *Canadian Medical Association Journal* 16, 820-823.

Riley, G. 1981. *Stuttering Prediction Instrument For Young Children*. Tigard, OR: C.C. Publications.

Riley, G. & Riley, J. 1983. Evaluation as a basis for intervention. In: D. Prins & R. Ingham (Eds.), *Treatment of Stuttering in Early Childhood: Methods and issues*.

References

San Diago: College-Hill Press.

Riley, G. & Riley, J. 1984. A component model for treating stuttering in children. In: M. Peins (Ed.), *Contemporary Approaches in Stuttering Therapy*. Boston, MA: Little Brown.

Riley, G. & Riley, J. 1985. *Oral Motor Assessment and Treatment*. Tigard, OR: C.C. Publications.

Rosch, E., Mervis, C., Gay, W., Boyes-Braem, P., & Johnson, D. 1976. Basic objects in natural categories. *Cognitive Psychology* 8, 382-439.

Rosenfield, D.B. & Nudelman, H.B. 1987. Neuropsychological models of speech dysfluency. In: L. Rustin, H. Purser & D. Rowley (Eds.), *Progress in the Treatment of Fluency Disorders*. London: Taylor & Francis.

Rustin, L. 1984. Intensive treatment models for adolescent stuttering: a comparison of social skills training and speech fluency techniques. Unpublished M.Phil Thesis, Leicester Polytechnic, UK.

Rustin, L. 1987a. *Assessment and Therapy Programme for Disfluent Children*. Windsor: NFER-NELSON

Rustin, L. 1987b. The treatment of childhood dysfluency through active parental involvement. In: L. Rustin; H. Purser & D. Rowley (Eds.), *Progress in the Treatment of Fluency Disorders*. London: Taylor & Francis.

Rustin, L. & Cook, F. 1983. Intervention procedures for the disfluent child. In: P. Dalton (Ed.), *Approaches to the Treatment of Stuttering*. London: Croom Helm.

Rustin, L. & Kuhr, A. l989. *Social Skills and the Speech Impaired*. London: Taylor & Francis.

Rustin, L. & Purser, H. 1983. Intensive treatment models for adolescent stuttering: social skills versus speech techniques. *Proceedings of the XIX Congress of the IALP*, Edinburgh.

Ryan, B. l974. *Programmed Therapy for Stuttering in Children and Adults*. Springfield, Ill: Charles C. Thomas.

Ryan, B. l979. Stuttering in a framework of operant conditioning and programmed learning. In: H. Gregory (Ed.), *Controversies About Stuttering Therapy*. Baltimore: University Park Press.

Schwartz, H. 1987. Subgrouping young stutterers: a physiological perspective. In: H. Peters & W. Hulstijn (Eds.), *Speech Motor Dynamics in Stuttering*. New York: Springer-Verlag.

Schwartz, H. & Conture, E. 1988. Subgrouping young stutterers: preliminary behavioral perspectives. *Journal of Speech and Hearing Research* 31, 62-71.

Schwartz, M. 1974. The core of the stuttering block. *Journal of Speech and Hearing Disorders* 39, 169-177.

Shames, G. & Sherrick, C. 1963. A discussion of non-fluency and stuttering as operant behaviour. *Journal of Speech and Hearing Disorders* 28, 3-18.

Shatz, M. & Gelman, R. 1973. The Development of Communication Skills: Modifications in the Speech of Young Children as a Function of Listener.

Monographs of the Society for Research in Child Development 38, 5. (Serial No. 152).

Sheehan, J. 1958. Conflict theory of stuttering. In: J. Eisenson (Ed.), *Stuttering: A Symposium.* New York: Harper & Row.

Sheehan, J. l970 *Stuttering: Research and Therapy.* New York: Harper & Row.

Sheehan, J.G. 1975. Conflict theory and avoidance reduction therapy. In: J. Eisenson (Ed.), *Stuttering: a second symposium.* New York: Harper & Row.

Shine, R. 1980. *Systematic Fluency Training for Young Children.* CC Publications Inc.

Shine, R. 1984. Assessment and fluency training with the young stutterer. In M. Peins (Ed.), *Contemporary Approaches in Stuttering Therapy.* Boston, MA: Little Brown.

Starkweather, C. 1982. Stuttering and laryngeal behavior: A Review. Rockville, Maryland: *ASHA Monographs* 21.

Starkweather, C. 1987. Fluency and Stuttering. Englewood Cliffs, NJ: Prentice-Hall.

Starkweather, C., Aronson, J. & Amster, B. 1987. An approach to to the study of motor speech mechanisms. In L. Rustin, H. Purser & D. Rowley (Eds.), *Progress in the Treatment of Fluency Disorders.* London: Whurr.

Starkweather, C., Gottwald, S., & Halfond, M. 1989. *Stuttering Prevention. A clinical method.* Englewood Cliffs, NJ: Prentice-Hall.

Steer, M. 1937. Symptomatologies of young stutterers. *Journal of Speech Disorders* 2, 3-13.

Stocker, B. 1977. *The Stocker-Probe Technique.* Tulsa, OK: Modern Education Program.

Stephenson-Opsal, D., & Bernstein Ratner, N. 1988. Maternal speech rate modification and childhood stuttering. *Journal of Fluency Disorders* 13, 49-56.

Till, J., Reich, A., Dickey, S. & Seiber, J. 1983. Phonatory and manual reaction times of stuttering and nonstuttering children. *Journal of Speech and Hearing Research* 26, 171-180.

Travis, L. & Knott, J. (1936). Brain potentials from normal speakers and stutterers. *Journal of Psychology* 2, 137-50.

Travis, L. & Knott, J. 1937. Bilaterally recorded brain potentials from normal speakers and stutterers. *Journal of Speech Disorders* 2, 239-241.

Trower, P., Bryant, B. & Argyle, M. 1978. *Social Skills and Mental Health.* London: Methuen.

Vandell, D. & Wilson, K. 1987. Infants' interactions with mother, sibling, and peer: contrasts and relations between interaction systems. *Child Development* 58, 176-186.

Van Riper, C. 1971. *The Nature of Stuttering.* Englewood Cliffs, NJ: Prentice-Hall.

Van Riper, C. l973. *The Treatment of Stuttering.* Englewood Cliffs, NJ: Prentice-Hall.

Wall, M. & Meyers, S. 1984. *Clinical Management of Childhood Stuttering.* Baltimore: University Park Press.

Webster, R. l979. Empirical considerations regarding stuttering therapy. In: H. Gregory

(Ed.), *Controversies About Stuttering Therapy*. Baltimore: University Park Press.

Wells, G. 1985. *Language Development in the Pre-School Years*. Cambridge: Cambridge University Press.

Wender, P. 1971. *Minimal Brain Dysfunction in Children*. New York: Wiley.

Williams, D. 1957. A point of view about stuttering. *Journal of Speech and Hearing Disorders* 22, 390-397.

Williams, D. 1987. Emotional and environmental problems in stuttering. In: *Stuttering therapy: Prevention and intervention with children*. Memphis, TN: Speech Foundation of America.

Wingate, M. 1969. Sound and pattern in "artificial" fluency. *Journal of Speech and Hearing Research* 12, 677-86.

Wingate, M. 1970. Effect on stuttering of changes in audition. *Journal of Speech and Hearing Research* 13, 861-873.

Wingate, M. l976. *Stuttering: Theory and Treatment*. New York: Wiley.

Wood, D. 1986. In: H. Wood, A. Griffiths & C. Howarth (Eds.), *Teaching and Talking with Deaf Children*. London: Wiley.

Young, M. 1984. Identification of stuttering and stutterers. In: R. Curlee, & W. Perkins (Eds.), *Nature and Treatment of Stuttering: New Directions*. San Diego, CA: College-Hill Press.

Zebrowski, P. & Conture, E. 1989. Judgments of disfluency by mothers of stuttering and normally fluent children. *Journal of Speech and Hearing Research* 32, 625-634.

Zebrowski, P., Conture, E. & Cudahy, E. 1985. Acoustic analysis of young stutterers' fluency. *Journal of Fluency Disorders* 10, 173-192.

Index